PALEO DIET for ATHLETES

PALEO MEAL PLANS FOR ENDURANCE ATHLETES, STRENGTH TRAINING, AND FITNESS

Rockridge Press

CONTENTS

INTRODUCTION

If you're looking for a great way to clean up your diet and complement your workout plan, you've come to the right place. The Paleo diet is a wonderful approach to eating healthfully without sacrificing flavor or feeling deprived. You'll eat plenty of lean proteins and quality carbohydrates that will help you maximize the benefits of every single training session. You'll also skip the gluten and low-quality, processed carbs associated with many "training diets." Instead, you'll opt for natural foods that provide long-term energy and promote muscle repair and growth.

It's pretty much a given that without proper nutrition, you'll never be able to gain the strength and endurance needed for training to maximum capacity. The problem is, with so many diets and magic pills out there, it's nearly impossible to sift through them all to find one that will be effective long-term. The key is to go with simplicity and common sense—both hallmarks of the Paleo diet.

Whether you're training for a marathon, working to build lean muscle, attempting to lose weight, or just trying to stay fit and healthy, the Paleo diet makes for an easy, delicious component of a healthful lifestyle. Throughout the pages of this book, you will learn what constitutes the Paleo diet and why it's a great plan to help you meet your fitness goals. You'll also find a variety of appetizing recipes arranged in meal plans designed specifically for your needs.

Without further ado, let's learn how to eat caveman-style!

SECTION ONE

What Is a Paleo Athlete?

(1)

THE BENEFITS OF PALEO FOR ATHLETES

Before delving into recipes and meal plans, it's important to understand the definition of the Paleo diet and how it can improve your athletic performance more than traditional diets that require carb-loading and fasting. After all, common misunderstanding is part of the reason it's so difficult for many to choose a healthful way to eat; you can't be expected to blindly follow a program when you don't know how and why it works!

What's the Theory Behind the Paleo Diet?

The Paleo diet isn't actually a diet in the traditional sense of the word. There are no calorie restrictions, and you're welcome to eat as much as you want anytime that you're hungry. The Paleo diet is more of a lifestyle. Of course, since the focus of this book is on how to best feed your body for athletic performance, the concentration will be at least somewhat on quantities of food as well as types, but in general, the typical Paleo eater isn't calorie restricted.

Also known as the caveman diet and the Stone Age diet, the Paleo diet is based on the premise that there are foods that are optimal for our bodies and others that are less so. Our bodies haven't altered much in the last ten thousand years or so, but the way we eat *has.* For eons, humans survived on basic foods such as lean proteins, fruits, vegetables, nuts, and seeds that could be hunted or gathered.

Our bodies were well adapted to these types of foods—then BAM! The agricultural age hit, and then the industrial revolution began in the late eighteenth century, introducing refined sugars and processed grains to the civilized world. Our diets transformed from whole, natural, foraged foods to one based largely on processed grains, legumes, and dairy. In the scheme of things, ten thousand years is only a blink in time, and our bodies haven't yet adapted to this change in eating.

In an interesting side note, the agricultural revolution didn't just change our diets; it also changed us from a species of constantly active hunters and gatherers to a more sedentary people who stayed in one place and worked in spurts. This change is also noteworthy from the standpoint that digestion and exercise go hand in hand.

What Is the Paleo Diet?

As noted above, the industrial revolution didn't just change the way we eat, it turned us into people who no longer had to remain active to survive. Consequently, diseases such as obesity, diabetes, heart disease, and various gastric disorders began to explode to near epidemic proportions. These diseases, often referred to as diseases of affluence, became so prevalent that a gastroenterologist named Walter L. Voegtlin made the connection between these conditions and the change in diet.

In an effort to help his patients, he recreated a diet based upon his belief that our bodies simply had not adapted to eating refined, processed foods. Lo and behold, a large majority of his GI patients showed significant improvement once they switched back to the hunter-gatherer style of eating, and the Paleo diet was born.

Why Is Paleo-Style Eating Better Than Traditional Carb-Loading?

Many people use the terms "fitness" and "health" interchangeably, but one does not necessarily equate to the other. For instance, how many athletes have tragically died from undiagnosed heart disease or complications caused by poor diet, performance-enhancing drugs, or just flat-out bad luck? Those people were likely extremely fit, but they most certainly weren't as healthy as they could have been. It seems pretty obvious that your goal should be to achieve both health and fitness, and the Paleo diet can help you accomplish this.

Why Traditional Carb-Loading Isn't the Best Way to Prepare

The vast majority of traditional training meal plans will load you up with breads, pastas, and other simple carbohydrates in the last few hours leading up to a big competition. The idea is that simple carbs are easily converted into energy that your body can use to keep you going; however, this theory has some holes in it.

First, simple carbs do provide quick energy, but the key word here is "quick." Like a sparkler on the Fourth of July, your energy burns fast and hot but fizzles out fairly rapidly—then you crash. That's not exactly ideal when you need to continue on for several hours. Even though you'll most likely reload at some point, it's better to have a sustained energy source as well as a quick one.

Another issue with traditional carbs from pastas and breads is *gluten*, which is a protein found in grains that can cause different levels of gastric distress in many people. Gluten isn't the only problematic component of grains, either. Certain ingredients in grains can actually prevent your body from absorbing valuable nutrients from the fruits and vegetables you eat. Carb-loading with grains simply isn't the ideal way to eat if you're trying to prepare properly for an athletic event.

So How Does the Paleo Diet Get You Ready to Roll?

Right out of the gate, you're going to be healthier if you've been living the Paleo athlete's lifestyle. You'll be free of toxins and the garbage your body can't digest. Your digestive tract will be clean and your circulatory system healthier so you can efficiently transport oxygen throughout your body. Physiologically, your body will be the well-oiled machine it needs to be heading into competition.

Prior to a race, match, etc. of any kind, you're going to be eating foods that are not only rich in complex carbohydrates, but also contain healthful amounts of protein that will provide sustained energy to get you through your event. When you combine your increased health and fitness with the proper fuel your body needs to efficiently create both quick and long-term energy, the Paleo diet is, without a doubt, the best way to go.

How Does the Paleo Diet Aid Athletic Performance?

High levels of exercise are extremely stressful to your body, especially if you're not nourishing it properly. *Acidosis* (the accumulation of lactic acid in muscles) that occurs during extreme exercise, damages bones and suppresses the immune system, while inflammation from tissue damage can interfere with healing and even breathing. Intense exercise can also drain your body of valuable minerals it needs for survival.

The foods you eat on the Paleo diet directly aid in all these areas, making the diet ideal for athletes. Here are just a few ways in which eating caveman style can improve your health and performance:

- Lean meats, especially lean red meats, provide essential amino acids known as *branch chain amino acids* (BCAAs), which are the building blocks of protein. Protein is, of course, the building block of muscle. The Paleo diet encourages regular consumption of high-quality, lean meat.

- When you sweat, you lose trace minerals that are essential to bodily functions. Your body needs to maintain the correct electrolyte balance, and the foods promoted by the Paleo diet are excellent sources of minerals.

- The Paleo diet helps balance your omega-3 and omega-6 fatty-acid ratio. Though both of these fatty acids are necessary for your survival, you should eat them in about equal amounts. However, modern diets tend to provide an inordinate amount of omega-6s and an insufficient amount of omega-3s. The Paleo diet encourages consumption of fish and other foods rich in omega-3s, while decreasing the amount of omega-6-rich oils.

These are just a few of the many ways in which the Paleo diet can aid your athletic performance. Throughout the rest of this book, you'll learn even more ways that eating Stone Age style will promote health and help you take your fitness goals to the next level. Whether you just want to be healthier and fitter, or you'd like to compete in the next Ironman Triathlon, Paleo-style eating will help you achieve that.

(2)

PALEO FOR ATHLETES OF ALL ABILITIES

Because the Paleo diet is a lifestyle, you don't have to be an extreme athlete to benefit from it. As a matter of fact, it's important to keep in mind that the diet was created by a gastroenterologist in order to help restore his patients' health. The Paleo diet is beneficial to athletes of all levels primarily because it promotes general health, which in turn helps your body perform at optimum capacity.

You Don't Need to Be an Olympian to Benefit from These Plans

The beautiful thing about modifying a healthful diet to complement your physical fitness plan is that you're just increasing and manipulating the amount of nutrients you consume. This means you're not filling your body up with chemicals or performance-enhancing drugs that damage your organs and detract from your overall health.

What may seem incredibly intense to you may actually be effortless to someone else, but that doesn't make it any less taxing to your body. If you're sweating and experiencing muscle burn from trotting around the block, your body is experiencing as much trauma as a person who has to run full speed uphill to break a sweat. You need to fuel your body to replace the lost minerals and fluids, as well as provide the BCAAs and other nutrients required to repair and rebuild.

For these reasons, the plans you'll find here weren't written exclusively for Olympians and super-athletes. If you're working hard simply to get fit and improve your health, you're still putting your body under stress, and you need to nourish it appropriately. The following recipes and plans are therefore just as applicable to you as they are to extreme athletes.

Eating Paleo Style to Reach a Healthful Weight

If you've ever fought the weight-loss battle, you've no doubt been told that you need to eat a low-fat, low-calorie diet in order to shed the pounds. Well, guess what! That's not the best way to go about it, especially if you want to keep the weight off permanently. Traditional weight-loss plans are bad for a couple of reasons:

- You may lose the weight, but you're not going to live the rest of your life depriving yourself of food simply to maintain your new weight. This is one of the main reasons that people yo-yo.

- Your body needs good fats in order to stay healthy. Categorically eliminating them deprives your body of essential vitamins and nutrients, including brain-healthful omega-3s.

- You're still permitted to eat processed, refined foods generally considered healthful as long as you don't consume more than your allotted calories for the day. You're not learning to eat properly for good health and long-term weight loss; you're just learning how to lose weight short-term.

By switching to the Paleo lifestyle, you're not going to feel deprived. Because vegetables and lean meats are naturally low in calories, yet high in fiber and nutrients, you can eat them until you're full anytime you feel hungry and still lose weight. Fruits and nuts are higher in calories and need to be eaten in moderation, but there's nothing better for a sweet tooth than a handful of strawberries or some cantaloupe.

Since you're eating healthful foods and avoiding processed foods and toxic chemicals, your body will naturally cleanse itself so that it can function optimally, which will also help you meet your weight-loss goals. Then, once you reach your goal weight, maintaining that weight will be a piece of, er...watermelon, because you'll already know how to eat well.

Maintaining a Healthful Weight with the Paleo Diet

Chances are good that once you start following the Paleo diet, you're going to lose weight if you're carrying around a few extra pounds, even if you're not trying, and maintaining a healthful weight won't be such a struggle either. Tweaking your weight is actually fairly simple, because you're eating natural foods and skipping the high-calorie, nutrient-poor foods that are a traditional part of a Western diet.

The fiber and nutrient content of the foods you'll be eating will keep you feeling fuller longer, and once you get past your sugar addiction, you won't crave food just for the sake of eating. You'll reach a point where you'll feel hungry when it's actually time to eat instead of simply having the munchies, caused by a sugar addiction. That makes it easier to maintain a healthful weight as well.

Finally, if you find your weight creeping up, simply cut back a bit on the higher-calorie fruits, nuts, and red meats, and increase your vegetable, leaner meat, and low-glycemic fruit intake. Once your life isn't centered on eating, your weight will no longer be such a struggle, and you'll find it's pretty simple to maintain a healthful weight.

Now that you know the basics of the Paleo diet, let's move forward and discuss some meal plans that will help get you through each phase of your training.

SECTION TWO
Endurance Meal Plans

3

AN INTRODUCTION TO ENDURANCE MEAL PLANS FOR PALEO ATHLETES

If you're an athlete who regularly participates in endurance events, you understand the value of *glycogen* availability. Simply stated, your body converts carbohydrates into glucose, which it uses as its primary source of energy. If you have more glucose in your bloodstream than your body can utilize immediately, it's converted into glycogen and stored for use later.

If you don't have enough glucose in your system or glycogen stored, the next most usable source of energy is fat. If you don't have enough fat, your body will turn to protein, but your body typically doesn't use it as efficiently as carbs or fat. Also, when you're working your muscles regularly and vigorously, protein is necessary for muscle repair and rebuilding, but your body will use protein for this only if it doesn't need it for energy. As you can see, adequate amounts of glycogen are imperative for an endurance athlete for more reasons than one.

Unfortunately, popular practice is to load up on simple carbs and grains in order to build up a store of glycogen. There are numerous reasons why this isn't the best way to prepare your body properly for endurance events. First, your body needs more than just carbs to be healthy and function optimally even under normal circumstances. This is doubly true if you're going to place extra stress on it such as extended, vigorous exercise, but there are very few nutrients in simple carbohydrates, breads, and pastas.

Another reason why loading up on grains prior to endurance events isn't optimal is because grains contain gluten as well as ingredients that actually interfere with nutrient absorption. Just to clarify, the most accepted way to prepare your body for a major athletic event is to load up on foods that have no nutritional value, may cause stomach and GI upset, and make it more difficult for your body to absorb the nutrients it needs to recover properly. If this doesn't make any sense to you, keep reading, because the solution is here!

How Paleo Benefits Athletes in Endurance Sports

If you talk to a Paleo athlete who participates in any kind of endurance sport, you're going to get a litany of reasons why they believe their performances have improved since changing to the caveman style of eating. The benefits of eating Paleo can be applied to several different aspects of endurance sports in particular, simply because it's a healthier way of eating.

Your Body Is Healthy

As already discussed, there's an enormous difference between being fit and being healthy, but Paleo athletes give just as much weight to one as the other. It's a proven fact that people who eat lots of fruits and vegetables, healthful fats, and quality proteins have a lower risk of heart disease, diabetes, and other diseases of affluence. The benefits of a healthy circulatory system and heart can't be understated when you're an endurance athlete.

Since the Paleo diet is naturally low in simple carbohydrates, the body is accustomed to burning fat as fuel and can easily achieve that during performance. Also, Paleo foods are much higher in micronutrients than traditional endurance athletes' diets, so the body recovers faster and more effectively.

A Healthy GI System

Gas, bloating, fatigue, and that heavy feeling that many of us feel from eating breads and pastas are unpleasant even if you have nothing better to do than lie around the house in front of the television. If you're preparing for an endurance event, however, it can be nearly crippling. Nothing pads your time like stopping to use the restroom because your stomach is upset.

According to statistics, about 1-percent of people are sensitive to gluten and experience at least mild GI upset after consuming it. If those are the documented numbers, imagine how many people just write the symptoms off without any knowledge of the problem. The Paleo diet is naturally gluten free, so you won't need to concern yourself about any of this—all of the foods you'll be eating are easy to digest.

Fruits and Vegetables Provide Quality Carbs

Simple carbohydrates, aka sugars, are composed of only a couple of molecules and have no fiber or nutrients that need to be extracted, so your body converts them quickly and easily into glucose. They are nearly instant sources of energy, but because they're so easily consumed by your body's "furnace," the energy doesn't last.

Grains are complex carbs, but the gluten and lack of substantial nutrients make them less than ideal as sustained energy sources, too.

Fruits and vegetables, on the other hand, are complex carbohydrates rich in vitamins and minerals that work to keep you healthy and energized throughout your endurance event. Because they're also full of fiber, your body has to work harder to break down the carbohydrates, providing a source of energy that lasts as long as hours. All the while, your body is using the minerals and nutrients to keep running in other ways as well.

If you'd like a good visual, think of simple carbohydrates and grains as a firecracker. You light the fuse, it burns down quickly, you get the bang, and the process is over. Now think of fruits and vegetables as a candle: You light the wick, and it slowly burns off the wax around it to provide light for several hours. The wax is the fiber and nutrients that surround the carbs and make digestion a slow, steady process. You're still getting the energy—you're just receiving it in a steady supply instead of in one big bang.

Paleo Food List for Endurance Athletes

Unlike some typical endurance food plans, eating Paleo style doesn't focus just on carb-loading, because if you want sustained energy to help keep you from fizzling out before your event is over, it's a good idea to incorporate some fat and protein as well. The inclusion of protein really helps give your body a head start on recovery as well, and can help keep you safe from injury. Two other components you're going to need throughout your performance are salt and water.

Your macronutrient need is going to change depending upon your individual body and the phase of preparation, exercise, or recovery that you happen to be in, but here's a grocery list of foods you should have on hand for before, during, and after your workout.

- Almond butter
- Apples, oranges, or other low-glycemic-load fruits
- Avocado

- Bananas
- Beef or venison jerky
- Boneless, skinless chicken breasts
- Broccoli, asparagus, Brussels sprouts, spinach, or your choice of leafy, green vegetables
- Dates
- Dried fruits, including pineapple, mango, banana chips, and raisins
- Egg-white protein powder (or your protein of choice)
- Eggs
- Extra-virgin olive oil
- Fruit juice, such as orange or tart cherry juice
- Green tea
- Kale
- Strawberries, blackberries, blueberries, or choice of berries
- Sweet potatoes
- Tart cherries
- Walnuts
- Watermelon or cantaloupe
- Wild-caught salmon
- Yams

This should be plenty to get you through your event from preparation through recovery. The rest of this section will examine what your body needs to prepare, perform, and recover; offer a selection of great recipes; and finish up with some sample meal plans to get you through your endurance event Paleo-style.

4

THE ENDURANCE PRE-WORKOUT PLAN

If you want to avoid running out of energy, aka "hitting the wall" or "running out of gas," it's imperative that you eat correctly, get plenty of rest, and hydrate well both on the day before your event and in the hours immediately leading up to it. One of the main benefits of preparing for your event Paleo-style is that you're not going to have that overly full, fatigued sensation that often accompanies carb-loading.

Another difference is that you're going to be eating a bit more protein and fat than a traditional endurance, pre-workout plan would dictate. This is because your body is already used to burning fat for energy, and it's going to need the protein to maintain muscle strength and health throughout your workout and with recovery afterward.

Many endurance athletes who have switched to the Paleo diet report three distinct advantages to leaving the traditional way of preparing for endurance exercise behind. These include:

- No digestive upset during exercise
- Longer, more stable energy
- Faster recovery

These advantages aren't just related to endurance training, either; in general, Paleo eaters report that digestive issues disappear and energy levels increase within a month or so after making the switch. It's important to note that the foods you eat throughout the different phases of endurance exercise may not be strictly Paleo, because the Stone Age man didn't exercise intensely for long periods of time. You'll still be incorporating fat and protein, but the typical percentages may be a bit skewed until after you recover.

The entire concept behind the Paleo lifestyle is to listen to what your body needs, so if you feel your body needs a shot of pure glucose to get you through a physically challenging event, then so be it. In a case such as this, however, note that there are foods that can fulfill this function without the side effects. Just as an aside, milk has the perfect combination of protein and carbs to give your body a great nutritional boost.

Is Dairy Paleo Friendly?

Strictly speaking, cheese and cow/goat milk are not Paleo, but many Paleo dieters do incorporate them. As long as you can tolerate dairy, there's nothing in cheese or milk that's bad for you if consumed in moderation—as long as you're okay with it, so are we.

The Importance of Proper Eating Before Endurance Exercise

You now understand how your body stores glucose as glycogen for later use. This is the first reason it's important to eat properly before endurance exercise, but it's not the only one. What you eat before you exercise determines both how you'll feel during the actual workout and how well you'll recover afterward. Simply eating isn't enough; you need to eat enough of the *right* foods.

If you've ever been exercising and felt the beginnings of nausea, hunger, cramps, brain fog, or fatigue, you know how these symptoms slow you down and impair your ability to perform at your peak. If you've ever had to stop because of muscle cramps, vomiting, or to use the restroom because of gastric distress, you probably know better than most how important it is to eat the right amounts of the correct foods before you work out.

While it's true that you need to store energy sources to get you through your workout, you also need to provide your body with the nutrients and minerals it needs to keep your body functioning properly while you're exercising. These include sodium and potassium as just two examples. You also need more macronutrients—the tools to build and repair muscle on the go.

If you eat properly before you exercise, you won't feel as sore or take as long to recover as you would if you didn't suitably prepare. It's even accurate to say that it's important to eat correctly before endurance exercise simply to make it safely through the event!

How Long Before a Workout Should I Eat?

Depending upon the duration of your activity, you need to start nutritionally preparing for it as early as the night before. As a matter of fact, you should start hydrating early the day before any endurance activity. Make sure to drink at least eight tall glasses of water throughout the day, as you're going to lose most of your stored fluids in the first couple of hours or sooner.

Traditionally, the "night before" meal consists of a visit to your favorite Italian restaurant. You gleefully gorge on your favorite pasta, accompanied by the rich, heavy bread, and finish the meal up with a big piece of tiramisu or whatever your dessert of choice may be. If you're feeling heavy, bloated, and lethargic just reading that, you're reading the right book!

Paleo athletes carb-load, but we do it using healthful carbs such as sweet potatoes or yams. Kale is another nutrient-rich fuel source you may wish to include in your meal. It does have fiber, but if you'll think back to our conversation about complex carbs, you'll remember that a limited amount of fiber in your pre-workout meal is a good thing.

As discussed earlier, you should include a protein and fat source in your meal, too. Chicken breast or omega-rich salmon are both good choices. Though protein isn't necessarily a part of traditional endurance preparation, research shows that it's essential for both your performance and your health. Simply stated, your body can't perform or recover properly without it.

It's important to eat a good breakfast about two hours before the event, too, though you want to limit the fiber in this meal. You should also include starchy foods such as bananas or yams in your breakfast. A good choice for breakfast prior to an endurance event would be a banana and a couple of eggs or a smoothie made with egg protein, bananas, and yams. If you like milk, you may want to include some in your smoothie. If you can't eat two hours before the event, take in about two hundred calories ten minutes prior to the start of the event.

What Foods to Avoid Before a Workout

Just as there are foods you should incorporate before you exercise, there are also foods you should avoid. Let's touch on those briefly and then move on to the recipes.

Sugar, Honey, or Other Simple Carbohydrates

Although you may be told over and over to drink a sugary drink or eat a chocolate bar right before you work out, this can actually hinder your performance by dehydrating you and causing surges of insulin in your blood that can cause dizziness, nausea, or fatigue. Your body needs water to digest sugar, and the last thing you need to do is draw valuable water away from your tissues.

Soy-Based Proteins and Other Legumes

Paleo people don't eat soy-based foods or legumes of any sort. They're toxic to your body, and soy, in particular, can lead to numerous diseases and debilitating conditions. Although many endurance athletes eat soy as a protein source either in the form of tofu, soybeans, or protein powder, it's not a food that you should incorporate into your diet for any reason.

Refined or Processed Foods

Though pastas, breads, candy bars, high-sugar nutrition bars, and other processed foods are commonly used by endurance athletes, Paleo athletes eat only natural carbs. An exception to this may be made in the form of "gu" or other carb gels, but only as a last resort.

Grains

Paleo eaters don't eat grains because they're packed with gluten and antinutrients that actually prevent your body from absorbing vitamins and minerals from other foods. This includes corn, barley, oats, rice, wheat, and all cereals. It also includes grain-like seeds, such as quinoa and buckwheat.

Now that you know what to do, when to do it, and what to avoid, let's get to the recipes!

Recipes for Pre-Workout Fueling

One of the best things about Paleo eating is that there is never a need to sacrifice flavor even when you're in heavy training. Any successful athlete will tell you that diet is every bit as important as training, and if you enjoy your food, you're more likely to stick with it. With this in mind, the following recipes were created to be both delicious and nutritionally balanced enough to prepare your body for intense, extended exercise. We're sure that you'll love them as much as we do!

No-Fail Kale Salad

Kale is packed with vitamins, including A, K, and B6, and the minerals calcium and iron. It's also a great source of antioxidants that help protect your cells from oxidative stress. The walnuts in this recipe also provide your body with healthful fats that will help get you through your workout, while the oranges provide complex carbs to help you store glycogen.

- 1 tablespoon lemon juice
- 2 cups kale, chopped
- 1 tablespoon cilantro, chopped
- 2 tablespoons red onion, chopped
- 2 tablespoons walnuts, chopped
- ¼ cup orange wedges, quartered

Toss the lemon juice into the chopped kale and refrigerate for at least 2 hours so the citric acid starts to break down and tenderize the kale. Thirty minutes before serving, add the cilantro, so that the flavors will meld a bit.

Immediately before serving, remove from the fridge and add the onions, walnuts, and orange wedges.

Yields 2 servings.

Rosemary Lime Chicken

This luscious chicken recipe delivers as big on flavor as it does on nutrition. Chicken is a great source of usable protein, and the olive oil adds a nice boost of healthful fat as well as flavor. Toss in the herbs, and you've got a winner whether you're training or entertaining. With this dish under your belt, steady energy is a sure bet.

- 2 tablespoons fresh rosemary
- 2 cloves garlic
- ¼ teaspoon unprocessed sea salt
- ¼ teaspoon cracked black pepper
- 1 pinch crushed red pepper
- 1 tablespoon extra-virgin olive oil
- 2 boneless, skinless chicken breasts

Finely chop together the rosemary, garlic, salt, black pepper, and red pepper until nearly ground. Place in a small bowl with the olive oil to make a rub. If possible, let the mixture sit for a couple of hours to infuse the oil with flavor.

Preheat oven to 350 degrees F.

Marinate chicken in the oil-and-herb rub for at least 15 minutes.

Bake for 20–25 minutes or until juices run clear in your chicken.

Serve immediately.

Yields 2 servings.

Baked Yam Fries

Yams are the Paleo athlete's go-to carb of choice. They are a good source of minerals such as potassium, phosphorus, magnesium, selenium, zinc, and other nutrients that will help get you through an intense workout, and offer about 40 grams of carbs per 100-gram serving. And they taste great, too!

- 2 large yams
- 2 teaspoons extra-virgin olive oil or coconut oil
- ½ teaspoon unprocessed sea salt
- ½ teaspoon Italian seasoning

Preheat oven to 350 degrees F.

Slice the yams into French-fry-like strips, and place in a bowl.

Drizzle with oil and sprinkle the salt and Italian seasoning over the yams. Toss to coat and layer on an ungreased cookie sheet.

Bake for 25 minutes or until tender and of desired crispness.

Yields 2 servings.

Stone Age Omelet

Rich in protein, complex carbs, and omega-3 fatty acids, this omelet will keep your motor running long after your carb-loaded competitors have dropped out of the pack.

- 2 eggs
- 1 pinch unprocessed sea salt
- 1 pinch cracked black pepper

- ½ avocado, peeled, cored, and sliced
- 1 teaspoon cilantro, chopped
- 2 tablespoons tomato, chopped

Whisk the eggs together and add to a hot 6-inch nonstick skillet. Sprinkle salt and pepper over the egg and cook for about 2 minutes.

Add the avocado, cilantro, and tomato and fold the mixture in half. Cook for another minute or so and remove from skillet.

Yields 1 serving.

Yambanana Smoothie

Packed with complex carbs, protein, and vital nutrients, this smoothie is a great way to load up on nutrition a couple of hours before you begin exercising. The milk is optional, but the casein it contains helps slow down digestion, giving you a more sustained source of energy.

- 1 medium banana
- 1 medium yam, cooked
- 2 scoops of egg-white protein powder
- 1 cup milk, almond milk, or green tea

Add all ingredients to your blender, and mix until it's smooth. If you prefer it a bit chewy, don't mix it quite as long.

Yields 1 serving.

Fruity Green Go Juice

The combination of complex carbs, protein, nutrients, and healthful fats in this smoothie will work together to keep your energy levels up while helping your muscles recover as you go.

- 1 medium avocado, peeled and cored
- 1 medium banana
- 1 scoop egg-white protein powder
- 1 tablespoon almond butter
- ½ cup strawberries
- 1 cup fresh spinach
- ½ cup milk, almond milk, or green tea

Add all ingredients to your blender, and mix until it's smooth. Drink it 2 hours before you begin exercising.

Yields 1 serving.

Paleo Nutty Fruit and Cream

This recipe is delicious, filling, and will provide you with sustained energy that will do its part to get you to the top. The combination of protein, carbs, and healthful fat gets your body geared up and ready to go.

- ½ cup strawberries, sliced
- ½ cup blueberries
- 2 tablespoons raisins

- ½ cup almonds, sliced
- 1 cup almond milk

Add the strawberries and blueberries to a cereal bowl, and top with the raisins and almonds.

Pour the almond milk over the mixture and enjoy.

Yields 1 serving.

Remember that hydration is just as important to proper preparation as eating well, so don't forget to drink your water. The next chapter will discuss more about staying well hydrated, as well as share additional delicious ways to keep your body fueled Paleo-style during your workout. So read on!

(5)

THE ENDURANCE DURING-WORKOUT PLAN

Even the best pre-workout preparation will get you only so far before your body needs more fuel. At the very most, you'll be able to go ninety minutes or so without eating before you begin to conk out, but remember that the effects from food aren't instant. Even carbohydrate gels take a few minutes for your body to absorb, so you need to feed your body *before* you start to feel fatigued.

The same goes for hydration, though maintaining adequate fluid levels may perhaps be even more important. If you run out of calories, you're going to crash, become fatigued, or possibly become nauseated. If you become too dehydrated on the other hand, you can actually die. In the second part of this chapter, you will find answers to how often you need to hydrate and how much you should drink in order to maintain good health and promote peak athletic function. Also included is a recipe for a Paleo-friendly sports drink.

Fuel on the Go: Maintaining Your Energy

According to even the most die-hard Paleo eater, there's nothing wrong with breaching standard Paleo protocol by using "gu" or carbohydrate gels to keep your glucose levels up, but there are also viable alternatives to that if you don't want to reintroduce simple carbohydrates into your system. In short, there is no right or wrong way to fuel your body as long as you're doing what works for you. One of the Paleo diet's number-one principles is to listen to your body, because it will tell you exactly what it needs.

In order to determine how much you should eat, you need to know approximately how many calories you'll be burning per hour. A good rule of thumb is to shoot for 200–400 calories per hour adapted for consideration of body size and level of activity. If you're going to be exercising for less than an hour, you won't need to eat; just water will be fine. If you're going to be exercising for longer than that, you're going to need fuel. Eating every thirty minutes is a good goal to set.

You want to include foods composed of both readily available carbs, a little bit of fat, and some protein that will help your body rebuild even as you're exercising. Protein helps maintain your muscles, and if you have plenty of energy but your muscles are exhausted, you risk injury. The protein helps tremendously here. Some fiber is good, too, because it will prevent sugar spikes and crashes by slowing digestion.

Many Paleo athletes who opt for natural foods instead of carb gels swear by dates, as they're packed with sugar and are digested fairly quickly. They're also extremely portable and easy to eat on the run. Several recipes that follow incorporate dates and other "quick energy" sources also rich in nutrients, which will get you through to that big celebratory dinner!

Why Hydration Is So Important

Every single cell in your body contains water and depends upon proper hydration for good health and function; in fact, your body is about 60 percent water. Just a few of the functions to which water is vital include:

- Delivering nutrients to your tissues
- Removing waste from your cells
- Transporting oxygen to your cells
- Dissolving chemicals so that they may properly interact with each other
- Dissolving nutrients so that your body may use them
- Controlling body temperature
- Lubricating your intestines, around your organs, and in your stomach
- Balancing electrolyte and pH

And this is just the tip of the iceberg. Though you can theoretically live up to several weeks without food, you can't last more than a few days without water. What's more, if you get even moderately dehydrated, your electrolytes or your pH can become unbalanced and cause life-threatening conditions. As you can see, staying hydrated isn't an option; it's critical to your survival.

In addition to the two obvious ways of eliminating water, urination and sweat, you also lose water during other bodily functions, including exhalation. In order to replace the fluid you lose while you're exercising, you have to drink. Since you're also losing sodium and other minerals while you're sweating, a good sports drink that replenishes your electrolytes is necessary. Here is a good schedule for water consumption to get hydrated prior to your event and stay hydrated while you're exercising.

- Drink eight large glasses of water the day before.
- Drink 16–24 ounces with your breakfast.
- Drink another 16 ounces two hours before you're due to begin.
- Drink 16 ounces thirty minutes before you start.
- Drink at least 4 ounces every fifteen minutes while you're exercising—just take a couple of large swallows on the fly.

If possible, drink cold water, because your body digests it more easily, and it also helps cool you down. If you don't drink enough water or replenish with a sports drink, you can experience nausea, cramps, brain fog, or headaches. As a matter of fact, if you begin to experience any of these symptoms, you should increase your water intake immediately. If you wait until you feel thirsty to drink, you're already in the first stages of dehydration, and your health and performance may be compromised. Drink before the feeling of thirst sets in.

Now that you know how often and how much you need to eat and drink, let's move on to the recipes!

Recipes for Fuel on the Go

Of course the goal behind these recipes was to create foods that were portable, easy to eat on the fly, and loaded with nutrients and a good ratio of carbs, fat, and protein. But even if you're eating only because you have to, there's no reason for it to be an unpleasant experience. So rest assured that each recipe that follows is every bit as delicious as it is nutritious and portable.

Date Bars

Dates are a great source of quick energy, and they're also packed with nutrients. The nuts provide a nice boost of healthful fats, and the banana provides potassium. The salt is also crucial to recovery because you lose sodium and other vital minerals when you sweat.

- 12 Medjool dates
- 1 small banana
- 1 cup dried sour cherries
- 2 tablespoons coconut oil
- ½ teaspoon unprocessed sea salt
- 1 cup walnuts

Combine all ingredients in your food processor and mix until it's thoroughly chopped and blended. It will probably turn into a big, gooey ball, but that's okay.

Spread the mixture out onto a cookie sheet and refrigerate for an hour.

Cut into 1 x 4–inch bars and wrap separately in plastic wrap, and refrigerate until you are ready to use.

Yields about 15 bars.

Paleo Jerky

You'll need a dehydrator for this recipe, but if you like the convenience and taste of this nutrient-rich snack, it's worth the investment. If purchasing jerky, make sure the ingredients include only meat and spices!

- 2 pounds beef, venison, elk, or other lean meat
- 1 cup coconut aminos
- 1 teaspoon garlic powder
- 1 teaspoon onion powder
- ½ teaspoon crushed red pepper or ¼ teaspoon cayenne pepper
- 1 teaspoon unprocessed sea salt
- 1 teaspoon cracked black pepper

Slice the meat as thinly as possible across the grain.

Add it to a large bowl, and pour the coconut aminos over the meat. Add the spices and stir until all of the meat is coated. Cover and marinate in the refrigerator for 24 hours, stirring every few hours.

Add to your dehydrator trays in a single layer, leaving plenty of room between each piece to allow for air circulation. Follow the directions for your dehydrator, drying the meat for the recommended amount of time. You'll know when it's done when you can bend the meat without visible moisture.

Store in a dry, airtight container.

Yields about 1 pound of jerky.

Paleo Endurance Trail Mix

This trail mix provides balanced nutrition that you can stick right in your pocket and eat by the handful every few minutes. It's a great source of minerals, vitamins, carbs, protein, and fat. If you're really industrious, make your own dried fruit. The only problem will be keeping the kids out of it until your event!

- ½ cup dried pineapples
- ½ cup dried mangos
- ½ cup dates
- ½ cup almonds
- ½ cup coconut flakes
- ½ cup dried bananas
- ½ cup jerky, shredded into small pieces
- 1 teaspoon unprocessed sea salt

Combine all ingredients in a bowl and toss to combine.

Store in an airtight container until you're ready to eat. On the day of your endurance event, place a portion into a baggie to carry with you. Snack steadily on it every few minutes.

Yields 3½ cups.

Tropical Fruit Leather

This is a bit of a twist on the ever-popular fruit rolls kids love, except this version isn't packed with sugar. You can use just about any fruit you like for your leather. For this one, we opted for a tropical feel. It's a great source of carbs and vital nutrients and is easy to eat on the go. The almonds give it a bit of fat and protein to provide you with sustained energy. You'll need a food dehydrator for this recipe.

- 1 cup ripe mango, cored and skinned
- 1 cup fresh pineapple chunks
- 1 cup coconut flakes
- 1 cup almonds

Add all the ingredients to your food processor, and blend until smooth.

Spread the mixture thinly onto the fruit leather tray that came with your food dehydrator.

Dry as directed, slice into 6-inch-wide strips, and roll up.

Store in an airtight container.

Yields approximately 12 roll-ups.

Yambanana Nut Muffins

These delicious, nutritious muffins are made with a great carb/fat/protein ratio. The fiber they contain will keep you going till the finish line!

- 1 medium yam, baked until soft, then peeled
- 1 medium banana
- ½ cup almond flour
- 1 teaspoon pumpkin pie seasoning
- ½ teaspoon unprocessed sea salt
- ¼ teaspoon baking soda
- 1 teaspoon baking powder
- 2 tablespoons honey
- 3 eggs
- ⅓ cup coconut oil
- 1 teaspoon vanilla
- ½ cup walnuts, chopped

Preheat oven to 350 degrees F.

Puree the yam and the banana together in a blender, and then add all the dry ingredients except the walnuts.

Mix until blended and add the honey, eggs, oil, and vanilla. Blend until smooth, and then add the walnuts. Stir until they're mixed through.

Fill cupcake papers or greased muffin tins halfway up.

Bake until a toothpick inserted in the middle comes out clean. Start checking at 25 minutes.

Yields 12 muffins.

Tuna Apple Sammies

These little delights are a sweet, Paleo take on a traditional tuna sandwich. Again, the ratio of carbs, healthful fats, and protein provides steady energy while helping to protect your muscles.

- 1 (6-ounce) can albacore tuna
- 1 boiled egg, sliced
- ½ avocado, peeled, cored, and diced
- 1 tablespoon diced mango
- ¼ teaspoon cilantro, chopped
- 1 teaspoon red onion, chopped
- 1 Fuji apple, cored and sliced into ¼-inch horizontal slices

Add all ingredients except the apple to a small bowl and mix well.

Add 1–2 tablespoons of tuna mixture to a slice of apple, and top with another slice. Eat like a sandwich.

Yields about 4 "sandwiches."

Paleo Sports Drink

You lose electrolytes when you sweat, and it's vital that you replenish them while you're working out in order to avoid cramps, fatigue, and even passing out or death. However, commercial sports drinks are full or sugars and preservatives. Here's a good natural alternative to help replenish your magnesium, potassium, sodium, and chloride.

- 8 ounces orange juice (may substitute 4 ounces lemon or lime juice)

- 8 ounces purified or filtered water (if using lemon or lime juice, increase to 10 ounces)
- 2 pinches unprocessed sea salt

Add all ingredients together in a 16-ounce cup and stir until salt is dissolved.

Drink a couple of large mouthfuls every 30 minutes as you exercise.

Yields 16 ounces.

Any of these recipes will do a wonderful job of keeping you energetic and moving until you finish your session. You'll also have a head start on muscle recovery because of your wise choice of foods. Now that you're all set to prepare for your event and maintain your energy levels throughout, let's talk about what you need to do at the end to help your body recover quickly and efficiently.

6

THE ENDURANCE POST-WORKOUT PLAN

Regardless of whether you've just bicycled twenty miles or finished your fourth Ironman Triathlon, your workout isn't over. As a matter of fact, how you care for your body in the minutes and hours following an intense, extended exercise session will have tremendous and lasting repercussions on both your immediate and long-term health.

Though nutrition and hydration are two key components of any post-workout recovery plan, endurance workouts are different from shorter exercise sessions and require a significantly different recovery strategy. The following pages will examine what you need to do to get your body back in prime shape and ready to go again.

What to Drink After Your Workout

One of the major differences that many Paleo athletes note is that since they've started living the caveman lifestyle, they recover more quickly and seem to suffer from fewer injuries than when they were following the standard, stuff-yourself-with-pasta endurance diet. Regardless of what the athlete eats, it's pretty much a given that the first thing that you need to do as soon as you jump off your bike, climb out of the pool, or cross the finish line is grab a recovery drink and start rehydrating.

Immediately After an Endurance Workout

In the first thirty minutes following your workout, it's imperative that you begin to rehydrate and give your body some protein so that it can rebuild and repair damaged muscle tissues. Even the strictest Paleo authorities say that a sports drink at this point is perfectly acceptable, because the typical Stone Age athlete didn't exercise the way that you just did, so this is one of the few situations that may call for a bit of deviation from Paleo standards.

You can also make your own sports drink that *is* Paleo. You'll find a recipe for a good one in the recipes section in the following pages. When preparing your drink, shoot for a carbohydrate/protein ration of 4–5:1 and 120–170 mg of sodium. Just so you know, that's about two pinches of salt. Use a protein that's as bio-available as possible; egg-white protein powder is optimal, but whey is the next best. Drink at least sixteen ounces of recovery drink in the first thirty minutes, as well as plenty of water over the next several hours.

Within the First Few Hours Post-Endurance Workout

Many athletes weigh themselves immediately before and after an endurance workout. Since you're losing fluids only, this is a good way to know how much water you've lost. A good rule of thumb is to drink 16–24 ounces of water for every pound that you lose in order to rehydrate in the first few hours after your workout.

A good sign that your body is finally adequately rehydrated is a return to normal amounts of pale urine and lack of thirst. Keep in mind though that if you're taking supplements, your urine may be darker than average for a few hours after you exercise. Basically, use your common sense. You know what your urine typically looks like. Assuming you normally drink enough, strive for "normal-for-you."

Don't Forget the Salt

Rehydration occurs fastest when you have adequate sodium levels. Since you lose large amounts of sodium when you sweat, you run the risk of *hyponatremia*, commonly referred to as water intoxication, if you drink large quantities of water without adding the sodium your water needs to absorb it. People who sweat profusely are at a higher risk for this condition, particularly those who lose significant amounts of salt while sweating. Sports drinks, either homemade or commercial, can help. Be careful that you're not drinking too much sugar though, because that can actually inhibit your rehydration efforts.

Refueling and Recovering After a Workout

As we've already covered, replenishing water, electrolytes, and protein should be your primary goal as soon as you've completed your event. You know how to replenish your water, and we've discussed sports drinks as another means of replenishing your electrolytes, but they aren't your only option. There are numerous foods that you can eat to balance your minerals out, too.

Focus first on salty snacks, since you lose more sodium than you do other electrolytes. Pickles, tomatoes, salted nuts, green olives, and crabmeat are all good sources of dietary sodium. You can also go with our Tropical Post-Workout Paleo Potion (see the following recipes), sipping on it alternately with water throughout the hours following your workout. Be careful, though, not to consume too much salt.

Though hydration is critical, it's not your only post-workout concern. Your post-workout drink should contain protein as well as sugar and electrolytes. That's your first step toward refueling your body, but you need to follow it up with proper nutrition, too.

For as many hours as your workout lasted, you need to continue to focus on carbs and quality proteins. Again, many athletes deviate from the Paleo style of eating during this period and eat pastas and breads, but you don't have to. If you don't want to reintroduce all of that processed food back into your diet, there are plenty of great, nutrient-dense Paleo options that will get you back on track. Here are some excellent foods that deliver carbs, electrolytes, and vital nutrients:

- Bananas
- Cantaloupe
- Kale and other leafy greens
- Milk
- Nuts
- Strawberries
- Sweet potatoes
- Yams

About an hour and a half to two hours after you finish exercising and have gotten a good start on rehydrating and repair, you need to eat a nutritious meal with plenty of complex carbs and healthful protein. See the following chapter for a few sample meals. After the initial post-workout meal, go back to your standard Paleo way of eating, which is basically, when you're hungry, you should eat. And always continue to hydrate well.

Recipes to Refuel and Recover

The following recipes are configured so you can mix and match them with other favorite dishes in order to refuel your body. The Paleo diet is ideal for this part of your workout because it consists entirely of foods packed with nutrients, including vitamins, minerals, and proteins. It meets your macronutrient needs regardless of your activity level, without compromising your health with processed foods and unhealthful fats.

Tropical Post-Workout Paleo Potion

This drink offers a great mix of fiber, carbs, protein, and electrolytes. It's also packed with antioxidants that can help your body fight the oxidizing damage caused by intense exercise. In a nutshell, it's great for you!

- 1 cup fresh pineapple juice
- ½ cup fresh strawberries
- ½ banana

- ½ cup frozen or 2 cups fresh spinach
- 2 pinches unprocessed sea salt
- 2 scoops egg-white protein powder

Combine all ingredients in your blender and blend.

The color is a bit odd, but once you taste it, you won't care what it looks like! Feel free to make modifications based upon your personal preferences—substitute the juice and the strawberries for your favorite juice and fresh fruit.

Yield 1 serving.

Southwest Grilled Salmon with Spicy Mango Salsa

Salmon is an excellent source of protein and healthful, omega-3 fatty acids, and the vegetables are a great source of nutrients and electrolytes. It's also so good that it may just become your go-to dish for recovery or entertaining!

- ½ cup tomatoes, chopped
- 1 teaspoon cilantro, chopped
- 1 tablespoon red onion, chopped
- 2 pinches unprocessed sea salt, divided
- 1 teaspoon jalapeno pepper, chopped
- 2 tablespoons chopped mango
- 1 lime, halved
- 1 tablespoon extra-virgin olive oil or coconut oil
- 2 (8-ounce) wild-caught salmon filets
- ¼ teaspoon cracked black pepper

Preheat oven to 400 degrees F.

In a small bowl, combine tomatoes, cilantro, red onion, 1 pinch sea salt, jalapeno pepper, and mango. Squeeze half of the lime over the mixture, and stir to combine. Refrigerate.

Grease a cookie sheet with a tablespoon of olive oil or coconut oil, and put the salmon filets on the sheet. Sprinkle the remaining salt and black pepper over the salmon, then squeeze the other half of the lime over them.

Bake for about 15 minutes or until fish flakes.

Divide the salsa over the top of the fish and serve immediately.

Yields 2 servings.

Garlic Chicken

Everybody loves chicken, but this dish will steal your heart as well as your stomach. It tastes like a comfort food and nourishes like a health food—truly the best of all worlds! Protein, antioxidants, and nutrients abound, so enjoy.

- 1 tablespoon garlic, minced
- 1 teaspoon basil, chopped
- 2 teaspoons extra-virgin olive oil
- 2 pinches unprocessed sea salt
- ¼ teaspoon cracked black pepper
- 2 boneless, skinless chicken breasts

Preheat oven to 350 degrees F.

Combine garlic, basil, olive oil, salt, and pepper in a small bowl. If possible, prepare an hour or so prior to cooking so the flavors can meld.

Rub the mix over the chicken breasts and place on an ungreased cookie sheet.

Bake 25 minutes or until juice runs clear.

Yields 2 servings.

Spinach Berry Salad

This is a power salad that contains everything you need to recover from your endurance workout. The spinach is packed with iron, chlorophyll, and vitamins; the nuts and dressing contribute healthful fats; and the berries give it a nice, sweet pop in addition to antioxidants and good carbs.

- ½ cup strawberries, sliced
- ½ cup walnuts, chopped
- ¼ cup feta cheese
- ½ small cucumber, diced
- 1 lemon, halved
- 4 cups fresh spinach

Combine all of the ingredients except for the spinach, squeezing half of the lemon into the mix.

Toss into the spinach and serve onto 2 plates. Garnish with remaining lemon.

Yields 2 servings.

Filet Mignon with Grilled Mushrooms and Onions

Sometimes nothing hits the spot quite like a nice, thick steak. Especially after an intense workout, lean, red meat is a great way to nourish your body and replenish lost protein. Get ready to really go caveman!

- ½ teaspoon garlic, minced
- 3 pinches unprocessed sea salt
- ½ teaspoon fresh basil, chopped
- ½ teaspoon red pepper, crushed
- ½ teaspoon oregano (fresh or dried)

- 2 (9-ounce) cuts of filet (or bigger if you'd like!)
- 1 tablespoon extra-virgin olive oil
- ¼ white onion, sliced and ringed
- 2 cups fresh mushrooms, sliced

Combine garlic, 2 pinches of the salt, basil, crushed red pepper, and oregano on a cutting board and mince together. Rub onto steaks and set aside. Allow to set for at least 20 minutes at room temperature.

Grill steaks in a skillet until they reach just below your desired temperature. Allow the steaks to rest in a warm place for 10 minutes.

In a medium sauté pan, heat the olive oil, and toss in the onions. Add the remaining pinch of salt, and sauté for about a minute and a half. Add the mushrooms and sauté for another 3 minutes or until veggies reach desired tenderness.

Plate your steaks and top them with the mushrooms and onions. Serve.

Yields 2 servings.

Venison Stew

Carbs, protein, and absolute deliciousness all in one bowl. Venison is a low-fat meat that is tender and juicy when prepared properly. The vegetables add antioxidants and vitamins that make this a great recovery dish. The best part is that you can toss this into the slow cooker and it will be ready when you get home!

- 2 pounds venison roast, cubed
- 3 cloves garlic, minced
- 2 red onions, quartered
- 1 pound baby carrots
- 1 pound fresh green beans
- 2 teaspoons unprocessed sea salt
- 1 tablespoon Italian seasoning
- 2 large sweet potatoes, cut into 1½-inch cubes
- 2 tablespoons coconut aminos
- 3 cups water

This is about as easy as it gets. Add all ingredients to your slow cooker, and stir to combine.

Cook on low for 10–12 hours or on high for 5–6 hours. Enjoy!

Yields 6 servings.

Grilled Watermelon and Ham Bites

Grilling watermelon gives it a unique flavor that plays really well with the savory quality of the ham and the creamy zestiness of the cheese. Plus it's a great combination of carbs and protein, so eat up!

- 2 (1-inch) slices of watermelon, quartered
- 1 tablespoon extra-virgin olive oil
- 1 teaspoon unprocessed sea salt

- 4 slices thin-sliced ham, halved
- ½ cup crumbled goat cheese (optional)
- 1 tablespoon coconut aminos or honey, (optional)

Preheat your grill to 350–400 degrees F and brush both sides of the watermelon with olive oil.

Place on grill and sprinkle salt lightly over it. Cook for 1 minute on each side.

Remove from heat and top with a slice of ham and a pinch of goat cheese. Drizzle with coconut aminos or honey and enjoy!

Yields 4 servings.

Now you know what you need to do to prepare for your endurance event, and how to stay hydrated and nourished throughout it. We also reviewed how to refuel your body when you've completed an event so that your body rebuilds and recovers appropriately. In the next chapter, you'll find a selection of sample meal plans coordinated specifically for your needs.

MEAL PLANS FOR SPECIFIC ENDURANCE SPORTS

Though your body's dietary energy needs are based more on the intensity and duration of your workout than type of activity, there are certainly major differences in how you consume that energy that are determined by your individual sport. For instance, biking is a relatively low-impact sport that can accommodate a fairly significant pre-workout meal without risk of stomach upset. Swimmers or runners, on the other hand, are at much higher risk of nausea or muscle cramps, and thus have different needs. This is why the following sample meal plans have been specified just for you!

Cycling Meal Plan

As with any endurance sport, bicycling requires stamina and staying power, but there are certain advantages that cyclists possess over other athletes. First, cycling involves smooth, rhythmic motions that aren't particularly jarring to your digestive system. This allows for a bit of latitude in pre-workout eating without too much risk of nausea.

The second advantage cyclists have is that they can carry food with them and actually eat in motion. This is a huge benefit, because no matter how well you prepare, your body can only store enough energy to get you through about two hours of strenuous activity. Fortunately, you have pockets, fanny packs, and backpacks!

Fueling Tip

Plan to consume at least 40 grams of carbs per hour, breaking that down however you'd like. Remember a constant stream of fuel is better than a one-lump fill-up, so try to eat at least every 30 minutes.

Night-Before Meal: Grilled Watermelon and Ham Bites, Rosemary Lime Chicken, and Baked Yam Fries

Breakfast 1–3 Hours Pre-Ride: Yambanana Nut Muffin, Stone Age Omelet, 1 cup cantaloupe, water

On the Go: Date Bars, Paleo Endurance Trail Mix, Tuna Apple Sammies, Paleo Sports Drink, water

Immediate Post-Workout Recovery: Tropical Post-Workout Paleo Potion, lots of water

Post-Recovery Meal: Southwest Grilled Salmon with Spicy Mango Salsa, Spinach Berry Salad, Baked Yam Fries

Throughout the evening and the rest of the following day, pay attention to what your body is telling you. If you feel hungry, be sure to eat and incorporate a good mix of protein and carbs so that your muscles can rebuild. Drink plenty of water before you actually get thirsty, and keep an eye on your weight and your urine. When everything is back to normal, congratulations! You've recovered and are ready to embark on your next adventure.

Hiking Meal Plan

Though hiking is a vigorous sport that requires proper training and diet, it places different demands on your body than higher-octane sports such as cycling, swimming, or running. Your calorie burn may be slower, depending upon where you're hiking and what you're carrying. Also, hikers tend to define long-distance hikes a bit differently than others might, so nutritional needs can be vastly different.

To a true hiker, a long-distance hike may be two hundred miles on the Appalachian Trail. For the sake of this plan, we're going to assume that the hike is no longer than a day's walk. The key is to take it a bit easier on breakfast, because you don't want a ton of heavy foods bogging you down.

Night-Before Meal: Rosemary Lime Chicken, No-Fail Kale Salad, baked yams with cinnamon, water

Breakfast 1–3 Hours Pre-Hike: Paleo Nutty Fruit and Cream, 2 scrambled eggs, water

On the Go: Paleo Jerky, Paleo Endurance Trail Mix, Date Bars, Paleo Sports Drink (if sweating), water

Immediate Post-Workout Recovery: Tropical Post-Workout Paleo Potion, water

Post-Recovery Meal: Garlic Chicken, Baked Yam Fries, fresh fruit bowl with mixed berries

Swimming Meal Plan

Swimming is an endurance sport that requires special dietary considerations for three reasons. First, it's an intense activity that burns a tremendous amount of calories. Also, you can't carry food with you like you can if you are cycling or hiking, nor are you near a readily accessible restroom. Finally, swimmers are prone to cramps, so you need to eat carefully in the hours preceding your event.

Night-Before Meal: Grilled Watermelon and Ham Bites, Rosemary Lime Chicken, Baked Yam Fries

Breakfast 1–3 Hours Pre-Swim: Yambanana Nut Muffin, 1 cup cantaloupe, water

On the Go: Date Bars, Jerky, Paleo Sports Drink, water (between breaks)

Immediate Post-Workout Recovery: Tropical Post-Workout Paleo Potion, lots of water

Post-Recovery Meal: Filet Mignon with Grilled Mushrooms and Onions, Spinach Berry Salad, Baked Yam Fries

Distance Running Meal Plan

Endurance running is challenging to your body and grueling to your system. Nutritionally, it's a delicate sport, because you'll burn a tremendous amount of calories, but you'll also be jarring your body in such a manner as to cause nausea if you eat too much or too heavily. Also, you're in danger of cramps due to the intensity of the workout and the electrolytes and water you'll lose through sweating. Here is a good sample meal plan to get you started and keep you going.

Night-Before Meal: Southwest Grilled Salmon with Spicy Mango Salsa, Spinach Berry Salad, Baked Yam Fries

Breakfast 1–3 Hours Pre-Run: Paleo Nutty Fruit and Cream, 1 cup cantaloupe, Fruity Green Go Juice

On the Go: Date Bars, Paleo Jerky, Paleo Sports Drink, water

Immediate Post-Workout Recovery: Tropical Post-Workout Paleo Potion, lots of water

Post-Recovery Meal: Grilled Watermelon and Ham Bites, Venison Stew, Spinach Berry Salad

These meal plans are simply suggestive starting points. The only way to create a meal plan that's perfect for you is to listen to your body's needs. If you have difficulty recovering from your first event, retrace your steps, and try something different next time. The keys to a successful endurance workout are to eat nutritious foods in the correct combination for your body and to stay hydrated.

The next section will explore how best to fuel your body for strength training and offer even more delicious recipes. Your next favorite Paleo recipe is only a couple of pages away!

SECTION THREE

Strength Meal Plans

8

AN INTRODUCTION TO STRENGTH-TRAINING MEAL PLANS FOR PALEO ATHLETES

If you've been strength training seriously for any amount of time, chances are good you're already eating a clean diet that's remarkably similar to a Paleo diet—you just didn't realize it. The reason you're so close is because your goal is to obtain optimum nutrition from every bite going into your mouth in order to get the most bang for every calorie. You also understand the importance of high-quality proteins. This section will delve into this a bit deeper and explain exactly how making the switch to a Paleo diet can really help you, whether you're bulking up or leaning out.

How Paleo Benefits Athletes in Strength Sports

We've already discussed how switching to a Paleo diet can help you by promoting good health, but there are other ways that make the caveman style of eating particularly suited to those of you who participate in strength sports. This is because your pre-competition or pre-workout diets are drastically different from those of endurance athletes, making your transition much easier.

Endurance athletes need to carb-load for up to three days prior to an event in order to store sufficient fuel to get their bodies through the intense, extended workout. Strength athletes, with the exception of competitive bodybuilders, don't need to drastically alter dietary habits, because the foods needed to prepare for an event or for an intense workout are basically the same ones that a strength athlete eats on a regular basis. The only real difference is a minor pre-workout and post-workout change in the carbohydrate-to-protein ratio.

Better Carbs

So, what if you could improve the quality of the carbs and protein that you were eating? It stands to reason that if you use better fuel, you're going to get better results. By trading your pre-workout rice and pasta for sweet potatoes, yams, or even white potatoes, you'll be getting more nutrients as well as fiber to help keep your insulin from spiking.

We touched briefly on the gastrointestinal benefits of giving up gluten in Chapter 3, but there are other benefits as well. All people are at least a little bit susceptible to the damage that gluten can cause, as gluten contains antinutrients that prevent proper mineral and protein absorption. This alone is obviously a bad thing for strength-training athletes who are trying to build muscle, but these antinutrients, namely phytates, lectins, and protease inhibitors, also produce an inflammatory response, which causes many people to retain water.

Water weight and puffiness, though certainly annoying, are only the tip of the iceberg when it comes to inflammation. It's also been causally linked to numerous diseases, including heart disease and cancer. Inflammation impairs your immune system as well, making it more difficult for your body to properly and quickly recover from aggressive training. If you can't recover properly, you're not going to build maximum muscle mass, so you're basically sabotaging yourself by eating grains, especially when vegetable alternatives offer so much more without the harmful side effects.

Overall, the Paleo diet offers healthier animal proteins that can help you build muscle more efficiently and lose fat faster.

Healthier Proteins

A chicken breast is a chicken breast is a chicken breast, right? You'd think so, but you'd be wrong. It's easy to look at packs of chicken breast in the grocery store and simply pick the one that costs the least, but those identical-looking pieces of meat are vastly different when you look at them a little closer.

Pick three chicken breasts that all appear to be exactly the same, but take a look:

- **Chicken Breast 1, nonorganic, mass-produced chicken breast:** This one was most likely grain-fed and injected with growth hormones. Meat is decontaminated with bleach and probably packed with a solution that contains such nasties as sodium, arsenic, chemical dyes, or hydrolyzed wheat protein. This actually has gluten in it.

- **Chicken Breast 2, free-range chicken breast:** This one's a bit tricky, because it sounds good, but the only obligation that farmers must meet in order to call the chicken "free-range" is to allow them access to the outdoors. They can still have chemicals, growth hormones, and other unhealthful gunk found in nonorganic meat.

- **Chicken Breast 3, certified organic chicken breast:** Organic meat must be allowed "access to the outside, direct sunlight, fresh air, and freedom of movement." That's straight from the USDA regulation on organic meats. They also must be raised without hormones, synthetic chemicals, or antibiotics.

Those three chicken breasts aren't looking quite so similar now, are they? Even organic chicken can be cleaned in bleach, so if it's at all possible, get your meat from local organic sources.

The nutritional value between organic and nonorganic chicken isn't really significant, but the differences between grain-fed and grass-fed beef are. In grass-fed cattle, the omega-3/omega-6 ratio is perfect at the recommended 1:1. In grain-fed beef, the ratio jumps to an unhealthful 1:6 due to the unhealthful fats in the grain. Too much omega-6 can cause an inflammatory response that suppresses your immune system and thus your recovery.

There's also the fact that cows have similar reactions to gluten that humans do, so the meat is affected that way as well.

In closing, you want your body to be able to recover efficiently and absorb nutrients, including protein, optimally. The Paleo diet helps you meet these needs better than a traditional diet that includes processed flours, wheat, legumes, and grain-fed meat. The grocery list discussed in Section 2 is applicable here as well, but this section will use it a bit differently. Let's move on now to discuss the best way to prepare for your workout.

9

THE STRENGTH PRE-WORKOUT PLAN

Because athletes who are training for strength events generally won't need energy for more than an hour or two, there's no need to eat during your workout like endurance athletes do, nor is there any real need to build up significant glycogen stores. In fact, you're probably already eating everything your body needs to successfully endure and recover, even from an intense, strength-training workout. What you do need to focus on is what you are putting into your body during the two to three hours leading up to your workout. This chapter will focus on that time period and present some recipes to make your pre-workout meal both healthful and delicious.

The Importance of Proper Eating Before Strength Exercise

As an athlete interested in strength-type workouts and activities, the mainstays of your diet are going to be lean, meat proteins and low-to-medium glycemic-load fruits and vegetables, with meat being the base. The reason for this is that you're tearing down and rebuilding muscle, and you're going to need the BCAAs (see Chapter 1) from the protein in the meat to achieve that. If you don't provide your body with the necessary protein to rebuild, you won't make any progress, and you may end up injured!

If you're going to be bulking up, chances are good you'll be eating more food than you've ever eaten in your life. Remember that one of the primary premises of the Paleo diet is to listen to your body and eat when you're hungry. Get ready: Once you start seriously strength training, you're going to be hungry every couple of hours. Best advice? Base your diet on meats, and fill it in with fruits and veggies.

Why are you going to be so hungry? Simple—when you work out, you're literally destroying muscle cells so your body can rebuild them bigger and better. That requires a ton of fuel, especially considering the extra calories your body is using to keep cool and the energy needed to lift weights! Plus don't forget that your body still needs to breathe, digest food, and all of the other functions that keep you alive.

Considering that your goal is often to gain muscle and lose fat in order to bulk up, the last thing you want to do is enter a calorie-deficit situation, so it's crucial that you eat plenty of the right types of foods and drink plenty of water.

Debunking a Paleo Myth

For some reason, people who haven't taken the time to investigate the Paleo diet thoroughly seem to believe the diet is low-carb and high-fat, which doesn't fit well with strength training. As you've seen, this simply isn't the case. Though fat is allowed, it should be healthful, unsaturated fats in moderate amounts, while carbs aren't restricted at all.

Getting Enough Carbs

If you talk to people who studiously avoid entering the Paleo camp, one of the first points they will try to make is that it doesn't provide you with enough calories to support heavy strength training. Again, this is untrue, though following one of the more modern versions of the diet that allows dairy and/or white potatoes certainly helps you consume more carbs while eating less. Both of these foods are hotly debated within Paleo circles, but the bottom line is that it's your decision.

One of the primary points to consider is that our ancestors worked their bodies differently than a strength-training athlete would; rather, they worked in short spurts. They ran, twisted, threw things, and bent over in spurts throughout the day, but they didn't perform hour-long work that required a ton of readily accessible calories.

If you take only one idea away from this book, let it be this: The Paleo diet is about fueling your body with clean, whole, easily digestible foods that promote health and don't cause sickness. If you feel the need (or simply want) to eat a potato, and you require the calories to keep your body functioning properly, then eat a potato. It's natural. It grows in the ground, and when consumed with other whole, natural, nutritious foods in moderate amounts, it's good for you.

Now that we've resolved the great potato controversy once and for all, consider using foods such as sweet potatoes, yams, dates, and dried fruits as high-carbohydrate food sources. You're getting loads more nutrients and just as many carbs as you would from a white potato.

How Long Before a Workout Should I Eat?

Food isn't instant energy; your body has to digest it and convert the carbohydrates, proteins, and fats into usable or storable form, and that takes time. In order to fuel your body properly for your workout, you need to eat a meal about two to three hours in advance. Though the time frame is the same as for an endurance athlete, the content of your meal is going to be significantly different because you're going to focus on protein as well as on quality carbohydrates and fat. Try to plan your pre-workout meal meals as follows:

- 25–35 percent lean protein
- 50–60 percent complex carbohydrate
- 15–20 percent healthy fat

If the majority of your workout is going to be aerobic, lean toward the higher percentage of carbohydrates and decrease the protein percentage. If your workout is going to be more anaerobic, build in a bit more protein and reduce carbs. Because the Paleo diet is individually adapted to meet your personal needs, it's hard to set a number of calories you should strive for: It all depends on how hard you're going to work and whether you're trying to bulk up or lean down. However, don't drop below a 500-calorie pre-workout meal, regardless of your goals—your body needs at least that much just to break even.

What Foods to Avoid Before a Workout

Nothing ruins a good, hard workout like nausea, vomiting, or hitting the wall ten minutes after you start sweating. In order to prevent this, there are some foods you should avoid within a few hours of heading to the gym. You want to eat foods that you know sit well and convert easily to energy or promote muscle healing.

Some of these you should never eat, but if you're going to fall off the wagon, pre-workout is not the time to do it. Most of the foods on this list are common sense but they bear repeating. This is, of course, a partial list, and some items on it may be perfectly fine for you. Only you know what your body can tolerate!

- Cream sauces
- Fried foods
- Gassy veggies, such as broccoli and cabbage
- High-protein, low-carb shakes or bars
- High-sugar foods, such as gels or juices
- Large amounts of fiber, such as a dinner salad
- Pizza
- Soda or other carbonated beverages
- Spices such as heavy basil, hot sauce, or curry
- Spicy foods, such as sausages

A great way to avoid getting sick during a strenuous workout is to be cautious. Stick with foods you know for a fact your body tolerates, and avoid those you've had problems with. If it makes you a bit queasy when you eat it on a date, you're really going to regret scarfing it down before lifting. Be smart and you'll be fine.

Now that you have an idea about what not to eat, here are some delicious recipes to gear you up for a blowout session!

Recipes for the Pre-Workout Plan

Remember that you get out of your body what you put into it! You need proper fuel to get through a good workout, and any good strength trainer will tell you that diet is at least half of the battle. If you're a hard gainer, you may want to double up on what you eat, but pre-workout may not be the time to do it. You want to eat enough prior to your workout to satiate your hunger and give you enough energy to last, but not so much that you feel ill. Find your comfort zone and stick to it—you can load up afterward.

If you can't eat a good meal an hour or so before you work out, at least opt for a snack such as fruit, because something is much better than nothing. Eat a good meal as soon after your workout as possible.

Savory Sweet Potato Hash Browns

These crispy potatoes hit the spot when you're looking for that salty, crunchy food to pair with your eggs. Sweet potatoes give you a nice boost of carbs along with vitamins and minerals, and the sea salt will help keep your electrolytes stable throughout your workout.

- 1 teaspoon coconut oil
- 1 medium sweet potato with skin, grated
- ½ teaspoon unprocessed sea salt
- 1 pinch cracked black pepper
- 1 pinch garlic powder

Preheat a medium skillet and melt coconut oil on medium heat.

Layer your potatoes evenly in the pan, sprinkle with salt, pepper, and garlic and stir.

Allow to cook until potatoes begin to brown, or about 2 minutes. Flip over and cook until brown on the other side, or about 2–3 minutes more.

Yields 1 serving.

Western Omelet Cups

These little bites are a great way to make your healthful breakfast portable. Mix and match the ingredients to suit your tastes, and combine them with the Savory Sweet Potato Hash Browns for a good combination of carbs and bio-available protein.

- 12 eggs
- ½ cup mushrooms, chopped
- ½ cup ham (uncured if possible)
- ½ cup green and red pepper blend
- ⅛ cup red onions, chopped
- ⅛ teaspoon unprocessed sea salt
- ⅛ teaspoon cracked black pepper

Preheat oven to 350 degrees F, and line 12 muffin tins with muffin papers.

Whisk eggs together in a bowl, and then add all of the remaining ingredients and stir.

Fill muffin cups up about three-quarters full, and bake for 25 minutes or until egg is set.

Yields 6 servings.

Paleo Waffles with Maple Syrup

These waffles are delicious and pack about 59 grams of carbs before you add the syrup. The maple syrup is absolutely Paleo and completely different than using refined sugar. It's rich in necessary carbs and also has a nice supply of minerals, including magnesium and potassium.

- 8 whole eggs
- ¼ cup coconut flour
- ¼ cup coconut oil
- ½ teaspoon vanilla extract
- ⅓ cup almond or coconut milk

- ½ teaspoon cinnamon
- ½ teaspoon baking soda
- ¼ teaspoon unprocessed sea salt
- ¼ cup pure organic maple syrup

Preheat waffle iron.

Whisk eggs well, and then add the remaining ingredients except the syrup. Stir well, but don't overmix, or your waffles will be tough.

Cook in waffle iron as directed.

Plate 2 waffles, and if you eat dairy, add a teaspoon of butter, if you like, along with 1 tablespoon of the maple syrup.

Yields 8 waffles.

Paleo Power Juice

Packed with antioxidants and good carbs, this juice is a delicious way to prepare for your workout without loading up on heavy fiber.

- 1 Fuji apple
- 3 carrots

- 2 large beets

Simply run all ingredients through your juicer and enjoy.

Yields 1 serving.

Stone Age Smoothie

This has a nice blend of fat, protein, and carbs, which will not only help get you through your workout, but get you started on the road to recovery. It's also packed with nutrients, including vitamins and minerals.

- 1 banana
- ½ avocado, peeled and cored
- ½ cup strawberries
- ½ cup dates
- 1 scoop egg-white protein powder
- ½ cup almond milk

Combine all ingredients in the blender, and blend until smooth.

Yields 1 serving.

Banana Carrot Nut Muffins

Nutritious, delicious, and totally Paleo, these muffins will keep you energized throughout your workout. Carrots and bananas offer medium-glycemic-load carbohydrates, and the dates are quick fuel. Plus, this is a great use for those ripe bananas.

- 2 ripe bananas
- 2 eggs
- 2 tablespoons coconut oil, melted
- ¾ cup carrots, shredded
- 1½ cups almond flour

- 1 teaspoon baking soda
- ½ teaspoon unprocessed sea salt
- 2 teaspoons cinnamon
- ½ cup dates, chopped
- ¼ cup pecans, chopped

Preheat oven to 350 degrees F.

In a large bowl, mash the bananas and combine eggs, oil, and carrots with them. Add flour, baking soda, salt, and cinnamon and stir well. Fold in dates and nuts.

Line 6 muffin cups with muffin papers and fill two-thirds full.

Bake for 25 minutes or until toothpick stuck in the middle comes out clean.

Yields 6 muffins.

Orange-Glazed Beets

If you're looking for concentrated carbs, this is a delicious side dish for your pre-workout plan—or any other meal! It's also packed with vitamins and minerals to help keep you going throughout your workout.

- 2 cups sliced beets
- ½ cup water
- 1 pinch unprocessed sea salt
- 1 pinch cracked black pepper
- 1 cup orange juice
- 1 teaspoon cloves

Preheat oven to 350 degrees F.

Place beets in a small loaf pan and add water, salt, and pepper, and cover.

Bake for 20 minutes or until beets are tender.

Put the juice and cloves in a small saucepan and reduce by half.

Remove from heat. When the beets are done, drain them, toss in the orange juice reduction, and serve.

Yields 1 serving.

(10)

THE STRENGTH POST-WORKOUT PLAN

We've said it before, but it bears repeating over and over until it sinks in: You have to refuel your body immediately after a vigorous workout in order to recover properly and start the muscle-rebuilding process. Replenishing after you train will keep you from getting sore, replace lost water and micronutrients, and restore depleted glycogen levels. Put this in caps, make it bold, and underline it: You can't skip your post-workout meal! In this chapter you'll learn a few tips on providing your body with what it needs to recover.

What to Drink After Your Exercise

Hydration before, during, and after your workout is key to building lean muscle mass, losing fat, and staying healthy. You've probably heard that before, and you do your best to stay hydrated, but here's a news flash that might help your motivation a bit.

The National Council on Strength and Fitness conducted a study on how hydration affects people before, during, and after resistance training. Insufficient hydration caused the release of stress hormones such as cortisol, norepinephrine, and epinephrine that triggered an enhanced catabolic response. Essentially, the body started to burn muscle for energy. Without getting too technical, even a modest lack of hydration affected core body temperature and blood plasma volume, which basically upset the entire apple cart.

The point here is that you need to drink plenty of water throughout your workout, at least sixteen ounces per hour. One of the best post-workout drinks that you could possibly consume is plain milk. It has a near-perfect protein-to-carbohydrate ratio; provides micronutrients such as sodium, potassium, and calcium; and the casein slows down the carbs so that they're absorbed slowly.

The key is to drink water until you're not thirsty anymore, and then drink a bit more. If you've lost a significant amount of fluid and salt from sweating, consider one of the Post-Workout Paleo Potions we've created here. There's one in the endurance post-workout section plus an additional one in this section—both are excellent for replenishing your electrolytes.

How to Tell if You're Hydrated

There are several ways to tell that you're getting enough water. If you're thirsty, you need to drink more, because thirst is a sign of dehydration. If your urine is pale yellow and plentiful, you're well hydrated. Finally, if you can pinch the skin on your arm or hand, and it slips back into place immediately, you're also sufficiently hydrated. Keep sipping all day every day, and you'll be just fine!

Refueling and Recovering After a Workout

If you drink a Paleo potion immediately after your workout, you're off to an excellent start, but you still need to eat a good meal within an hour or so, too. Incorporate a mix of lean proteins and healthful carbs, along with some good fats. In other words, eat a real meal! Because we're talking Paleo here, let your body tell you what it needs, and eat until you're full. Don't force yourself to eat more just because somebody said you should; when you feel full, your body is telling you it has all that it needs or can handle right then.

Here are some super-replenishing, healthful recipes to help you recover after a ripping training session or competition.

Recipes to Refuel and Recover

The key to proper recovery after an aggressive training session is to eat a sensible meal consisting of an equal blend of lean protein, complex carbohydrates, and good fats. The one difference between this meal and others is that in this case you may want to include a quick carb, such as some juice or a piece of high-glycemic-load fruit, so your body has something to start recovering with immediately. So go ahead and enjoy these recipes!

Berrylicious Post-Workout Paleo Potion

The berries in this drink give you a boost of antioxidants that work to protect you from oxidation, while the banana, spinach, milk, and salt provide you with electrolytes and micronutrients you need to recover.

- 1 cup fresh apple or cranberry juice
- ¼ cup fresh strawberries
- ¼ cup fresh raspberries
- ¼ cup fresh blueberries
- ½ banana
- ½ cup frozen or 2 cups fresh spinach
- ½ cup milk, almond milk, or water
- 2 pinches unprocessed sea salt
- 2 scoops egg-white protein powder

Simply add all ingredients except for the salt and protein powder to your blender, and pulse until pureed. Stir in the protein and salt, and enjoy.

Yields 1 serving.

Cajun Tilapia

This seasoned, slightly spicy tilapia is sure to please your taste buds as much as your metabolism. The spices, including garlic and cayenne, help keep your motor running, while the tilapia provides healthful fats and lean protein.

- 2 tablespoons garlic powder
- 2 tablespoons cayenne
- 3 tablespoons paprika
- 1 tablespoon cracked black pepper (you can use ground, too)
- 1 tablespoon onion powder
- 1½ tablespoons dried oregano
- 1 tablespoon dried thyme
- ½ tablespoon dried basil
- 2 tablespoons unprocessed sea salt
- 1 teaspoon crushed red pepper flakes
- 2 (4–6-ounce) tilapia filets
- Coconut or extra-virgin olive oil
- 2 lemon wedges

Preheat oven to 350 degrees F.

Gather all ingredients for the rub, and combine well in a small bowl. Reserve 2 teaspoons and store the rest in an airtight container. You've just made some amazing Cajun seasoning!

Rub 1 teaspoon of the seasoning on each filet, and place on a baking sheet sprayed with coconut oil or olive oil.

Bake for 15–20 minutes or until the fish flakes with a fork.

Plate and garnish with the lemon.

Yields 2 servings.

Talkin' Turkey Soup

This soup has a nice mix of protein and carbs and is filling enough to keep you going for a bit. The sodium in the broth helps you recover as well.

- 2 turkey breasts, chopped into 1-inch cubes
- 2 cups organic chicken broth
- 1 yam, cubed into bite-sized pieces
- 1 cup carrots, sliced
- 1 teaspoon cracked black pepper
- ½ cup kale, chopped
- Unprocessed sea salt to taste 1 cup water
- 1 cup celery, chopped

Sear your turkey lightly until it starts to brown.

Combine all ingredients except for the celery in a stock pot.

Bring to a simmer until yams and carrots begin to get tender, and then add the celery. Continue cooking until vegetables are tender and turkey is 100 percent cooked through.

Yields about 6 servings.

Nutty Chopped Salad

This is one of the freshest and quickest salads you'll ever prepare. Its tart-sweet dressing brings out the flavors in any vegetables, and you can use whatever greens you have on hand.

- 1 teaspoon honey
- 1 tablespoon lemon juice
- 2 cups mixed greens, chopped
- 1 tablespoon pine nuts
- 1 tablespoon tomatoes, diced
- 1 tablespoon cucumbers, diced
- 1 tablespoon red sweet pepper, diced
- 1 tablespoon red onion, diced
- 1 tablespoon avocado, peeled, cored, and sliced

Combine honey and lemon juice in a small bowl and set aside.

Mix together all other ingredients, toss with the honey-lemon mixture to coat, and enjoy.

Yields 1 serving.

Paleo Pesto Chicken

Sure, cave dwellers didn't have pesto, but this delectable paste will definitely add some spice to an otherwise ordinary chicken meal. If you prefer not to use cheese, that's okay—this recipe is just as delicious without it.

- ½ cup packed, fresh basil
- 1 tablespoon pine nuts
- 1 clove garlic
- 1 tablespoon pecorino cheese, grated

- 1 pinch unprocessed sea salt
- 1 pinch cracked black pepper
- 1 tablespoon extra-virgin olive oil
- 2 boneless, skinless chicken breasts

Preheat oven to 350 degrees F.

Place everything but the chicken in a food processor, and pulse to a paste.

Rub the pesto on the chicken, and bake on lightly oiled baking sheet for 20–25 minutes, or until chicken is done.

Yields 2 servings.

Kale Succotash

Kale is good for you no matter what health goals you have, and the sweet potatoes in this dish provide flavor as well as carbs. Add caramelized onions, and you have a real post-workout winner.

- 2 teaspoons extra-virgin olive oil
- ½ cup red onion, chopped
- 3 cloves garlic, chopped
- 1 cup cubed sweet potatoes
- 2 cups kale, roughly chopped with the stems and veins removed
- ½ cup chicken stock

Heat the olive oil in a medium skillet.

Add the onions, garlic, and sweet potatoes, and sauté until the vegetables start to soften, and then add the kale, and stir it all together.

Add the chicken stock and cover. Simmer on medium heat for 8–10 minutes, or until the kale is soft.

Yields 2 servings.

Mashed Cauliflower

If you're a mashed potato lover, then you'll most likely enjoy this. It's a great recovery food, because it has a significant amount of easily bio-available carbs.

- 2 cups cauliflower florets
- 1 tablespoon cow's milk or plain almond milk
- 1 pinch unprocessed sea salt
- 1 pinch cracked black pepper
- 1 teaspoon butter (optional)

Steam cauliflower until it's tender.

Place in bowl, add milk, salt, and pepper, and whisk with a mixer on medium speed until smooth.

Plate and add butter, if you'd like.

Yields 1 serving.

All of these recipes are great for your post-workout meal and taste terrific, too. There really is no reason why you can't eat a healthful, Paleo diet and maintain—or even improve—your appearance and performance as a strength-training athlete. In the following chapter, we'll look at way to bulk-up and lean-out. Chapter 12 ties it all together with meal plans for specific strength sports using all these delicious, nutritious recipes.

⑪

THE BULKING-UP AND LEANING-OUT PLAN

One of the many differences between endurance athletes and strength athletes is that endurance athletes train in basically the same manner year-round. If there's an off-season, they may slack off a bit and just work on maintenance, and then pick it back up a month or two before competitions start rolling around again.

Strength athletes, especially competitive-strength athletes, train in cycles because competing conditions require such a low body-fat percentage that you can't realistically maintain it year-round. Also, your body responds better when you're not aggressively training in the same manner constantly. Therefore, it's standard practice to train in cycles: bulking up and then leaning out right before a competition.

As you can imagine, this requires significantly different eating habits. During bulking-up phases, you're going to be eating large quantities of food. When you're leaning out, on the other hand, you're going to be calorie restricted because your goal is to reduce your body fat. Thankfully, when you're doing it Paleo-style, you'll still have plenty to eat because your calories are coming from lean proteins, fruits, and vegetables.

Since we're talking Paleo-style eating, you'll be eating when you're hungry, but you'll also be doing a bit more than that regardless of what phase of the cycle you're in. Because you're placing huge demands upon your body, you need to plan your meals accordingly. It may even be necessary for you to supplement what you eat in order to reach your goals, but generally it's possible to meet your needs simply by working and eating properly, if you're diligent. All of this will be covered in the next few paragraphs.

Eating to Bulk Up

If you're new to lifting, this is a term that you're going to be hearing frequently. All it means is that you're going to be eating more and training harder in order to build more muscle faster. That may sound simple, but it's not quite as easy as you might imagine. As we learn more about how the body works, smart lifters strive to eat smarter, not just in greater volume. There's a fine line between bulking up and becoming overweight, and that line is defined by what you eat, not how much. Fortunately, the Paleo diet offers a wide variety of foods that pack a huge nutritional punch without adding significant trans fats or empty calories.

There are several reasons why you may choose to bulk up:

- You just want to be bigger so you look good at the beach, etc.
- You're competing and want to move up a class
- You're just doing a bulking cycle, like many builders do for their winter cycle
- You play a competitive sport that requires strength, such as football or wrestling
- You're a hard gainer and want to build muscle

Your body is like a house: In order to add a second story, you'll need plenty of lumber. Also like a house, if you use low-quality materials, your end product won't look good or be structurally sound, at least not for long. The secret to bulking up properly without getting fat is to proportionally increase your healthful macronutrient intake. Translation? Eat more low-to-medium glycemic-load carbs, lean proteins, and healthful fats, and do it in a planned, controlled manner. Of course, you do have to take your training up a notch (or several notches, as the case may be), but you won't bulk up successfully without maintaining a healthful diet.

When Should I Bulk Up?

In order to really pack on clean-looking muscle, you need to be in decent shape with a fairly low body-fat percentage when you start your bulking-up program. If you have more than 10-percent body fat—a good way to tell: you can't see your abs—you need to diet and get down to where you can before considering a bulking-up program. You should at least be down to where you have a four-pack so you're starting from a point where your body is ready to pack on the muscle without padding up with fat.

Many bodybuilders believe that bulking up occurs more easily after you've been on a restrictive diet for a while, but to be truthful, the restrictive diet they follow is most likely nutrient-poor, so it's only logical that when their body is no longer being starved, it's going to respond positively by getting bigger.

Revolutionary Change of Plans

Unless your goal is to be fat, sick, and injured, ditch the idea of scarfing down fast food cheeseburgers after lifting massive amounts of weight until your arms are ready to fall off—it's a horrible idea. Remember that there's a huge difference between being physically fit and being healthy. It shouldn't have to be a to choice though: You can be both, and why wouldn't you want to?

There are some basics to bulking up healthfully. Your goal is to create a caloric surplus so your body can use the extra to recover and build with, but you want to take care you're not giving it so much excess that it's storing it as fat. You have physical limitations as well, since your body can digest only so much food at a time.

Because food requirements when you're bulking up will vary based upon your particular metabolism, weight, and workout, you'll have to calculate the exact amount you should be eating based upon your personal needs, but there are some general guidelines to get you started on the right path. Here are some pointers to help you successfully bulk up:

- **Lean Protein:** Protein, as you know, provides the basic building blocks of muscle. If you're not getting enough quality protein, you won't bulk up no matter how much you lift, nor will you recover properly. Shoot for 1–1.5 grams of lean protein per pound of body weight per day. Don't go too high, because as in most cases, too much of a good thing can be a bad thing; eating too much protein can damage your kidneys as well as cause other problems.

- **Complex Carbohydrates:** Simple carbohydrates really don't have any place in a strength-training regimen, because you aren't going to be working out long enough to burn through your energy stash as long as you're eating properly. Just like with protein, build 1–1.5 grams of carbs into your diet, and divide them so you're consuming about one-third of them in the morning and another one-third in your post-workout meal. Those are the times that your body absorbs and uses them optimally. Build the other one-third into your other meals, and make them fibrous so your digestive tract remains clean and ready to absorb more nutrients.

- **Healthful Fats:** About half of your brain is made of omega-3 fatty acids, and your body uses them as well for hormone production, disease prevention, and myriad of other necessary activities. Unlike unhealthful trans fats, Healthful unsaturated fats such as olive oil, coconut oil, almond butter, and avocado oil help prevent disease, build muscle, and promote brain function, and your body can't produce them—you have to eat them. Shoot for about three tablespoons per day, or 20 percent of your daily diet. There are nine calories in a gram of fat.

- **Water:** The biggest mistake you can make if you're trying to be healthy is to skip the water. About 60 percent of your body is water, and the part that isn't counts on the parts that are. Water lubricates your joints, flushes out fat and toxins, keeps all of your major organs functioning properly, and keeps your tissues healthy. You won't thrive long-term without proper hydration!

Now that you know the macronutrient breakdown, adapt it to your needs. Eat a wide range of foods to ensure you're getting all of the micronutrients you need as well. Divide your daily intake into at least five meals, preferably more, making sure that you eat plenty of carbs in your pre- and post-workout meals to make certain your body maintains adequate glycogen stores and can recover properly. Let's talk for a minute now about the leaning-out cycle that you'll likely experience if you're planning on competing, and then we'll move on to some amazing recipes!

Leaning Out

As with all fat-loss diets, leaning out involves creating a calorie deficit. Quite simply put, you lose weight when you burn more calories than you consume. The tricky thing about leaning out is that you have worked hard for all of that muscle and you don't want to lose it! Though every person who is trying to lose weight should concentrate on gaining muscle while losing fat, it's particularly important for strength trainers.

Unfortunately, old-school thinkers will use this time to ridiculously restrict their diets in order to strip fat off as quickly possible, but this is short-term, unhealthful thinking. Your goal should be to lose one to two pounds per week, and you need to use calipers, not scales, to measure your fat loss. If you're losing weight but the calipers show that you're not losing fat, then it's only logical that you're losing muscle. This means one of two things, or a combination of both: either you're not eating enough of the right foods, or you're not working out efficiently.

So What's the Dietary Secret to Stripping off Fat?

This is the most common question that people seeking to lean out inquire about the program. They see people carrying around huge jugs of water and green smoothies and wonder how on Earth they're ever going to get the hang of eating everything required. Well guess what the big secret is! The little-known fact to stripping off fat is simply to follow the same diet you do when bulking or maintaining—you just adjust the amounts.

Super-Secret Diet Tip for Leaning Out

Your macronutrient needs don't change whether you're bulking up or leaning out. You still need to eat proportional quantities of protein and carbs with an adequate amount of healthful fat. Follow the guidelines above, and if that seems confusing, think of it this way: Shoot for about 40 percent lean protein, 40 percent complex carbs, and 20 percent healthful fats—that's it!

Mapping It Out

You can't just stop eating when you're leaning out—your muscles need that nutrition. You probably already know exactly how many calories you're burning, so take that number and subtract 1,000, and that equals the number of calories per day you need to eat. If you burn roughly 2,000 calories per day just by existing (breathing, moving, walking, etc.), and you burn another 1,000 calories at the gym, you need to be consuming 2,000 calories per day in order to lose about 1.5 pounds per week. That's just an example, but you get the idea.

So here's the rundown:

- Use calipers to make sure that you're losing fat, not muscle
- Don't get crazy—you want to lose fat slowly in order to stay healthy

- Don't stop weight training, because you continue to burn fat for hours after you lift
- Use cardio as a way to create a calorie deficit
- Drink plenty of water!

That about covers what you need to do either to bulk up or lean out, so let's get on with the deliciousness!

Recipes for Bulking Up and Leaning Out

Because your macronutrient intake is going to be the same, just in reduced amounts, if you follow a healthful regimen such as the Paleo diet, the same foods will be useful for both phases. No matter what cycle you're currently focusing on, simply adjust the amounts you eat, and you'll be good to go.

Mediterranean Salmon

Packed with omega-3s and protein, salmon is a great addition to any training regimen. When you add in the spices and grill to perfection, you won't even know that you're being good.

- 1 tablespoon extra-virgin olive oil
- 1 teaspoon fresh cilantro, chopped
- 1 pinch unprocessed sea salt
- 1 pinch pink or cracked black pepper
- 1 clove garlic, minced
- ½ teaspoon ground cumin
- 2 (6-ounce) wild-caught salmon filets
- 2 lemon wedges

Add oil, cilantro, salt, pepper, garlic, and cumin to a small dish and combine. Brush over salmon filets, and allow to sit for at least 15 minutes.

Preheat grill to medium, and grill salmon about 5 minutes per side, depending upon thickness and how done you like your salmon.

Plate and garnish with the lemon wedge.

Yields 2 servings.

Nutty Kale-Stuffed Chicken Breast

This dish has it all. Pine nuts pack a huge, essential fatty-acid punch, while the chicken adds excellent lean protein, and the kale kicks in veggie carbs and a ton of micronutrients. The tang of the goat cheese puts the flavor of this dish totally over the top.

- 2 boneless, skinless chicken breasts
- 1 cup frozen kale, or fresh kale, blanched and chopped
- 1 tablespoon organic goat cheese
- 1 tablespoon pine nuts
- 1 pinch unprocessed sea salt
- 1 pinch cracked black pepper
- 2 teaspoons coconut oil

Preheat oven to 350 degrees F.

Clean chicken breasts and place on cutting board with the smooth side up. Slice a 2-inch slit in the middle of the breast and make it about ½-inch deep, then cut around inside the breast to form a pocket. Make a similar pocket on the second breast.

Combine kale, goat cheese, pine nuts, salt, and pepper, and stuff half the mixture into each pocket.

Brush with coconut oil and bake for 25 minutes or until chicken is done.

Yields 2 servings.

Yam with Mango Mix

If you're looking for a zesty, delicious side dish that's packed with readily available carbs, this is the dish for you. Perfect for your post-workout meal.

- 1 yam, chunked
- 1 teaspoon coconut oil
- 1 pinch unprocessed sea salt
- 1 pinch cracked black pepper
- 1 tablespoon mango, diced
- 1 tablespoon red onions
- ½ teaspoon cilantro

Preheat oven to 400 degrees F.

Put yams in a small baking dish, drizzle with the oil, salt, and pepper, and bake for 25 minutes or until yams are tender.

Combine mango, onion, and cilantro, and sprinkle over the yams when they're finished.

Yields 1 serving.

Egg-White Hash

This is a healthier take on a Western omelet. Packed with protein, it's a great way to start your day!

- ¼ cup pancetta, chopped
- ¼ cup green peppers, chopped
- ¼ cup red onions, diced
- 2 pinches unprocessed sea salt
- 1 pinch cracked black pepper
- 6 egg whites
- ¼ cup tomatoes, diced
- 1 teaspoon hot sauce (optional)

Sauté the pancetta, green peppers, and red onions in a medium skillet on medium heat until the pancetta crisps and onions are getting translucent.

Sprinkle on the salt and pepper, and add the egg whites and tomatoes. Stir together and cook until egg whites are done.

Plate and sprinkle with hot sauce if desired.

Yields 2 servings.

Best-Ever Beef Kabobs

Tender, juicy, and zesty, these kabobs are going to make you glad you're eating healthfully. Yet more proof that bulking up or leaning out doesn't have to taste unappetizing!

- ½ cup coconut aminos
- 1 teaspoon unprocessed sea salt
- 1 teaspoon cracked black pepper
- 1 clove garlic, minced
- ¼ teaspoon red pepper flakes
- ¼ teaspoon rosemary, chopped
- ¼ teaspoon basil, chopped

- 1 pound lean red meat, such as beef, venison, or bison, chunked into bite-sized cubes
- 1 red onion, peeled, cut in half horizontally, and quartered vertically
- 1 pack cherry tomatoes
- 2 green peppers, cut similarly to the onion

Mix together the first seven ingredients.

Add the meat to a large plastic zip bag, and pour the spice mixture over it. Marinate for at least 20 minutes—the longer the better.

Preheat the grill to medium-high when you're ready to make the kabobs.

Thread the meat, onions, tomatoes, and peppers onto your skewers.

Grill 1–3 minutes on each of the 4 sides, or until your steak reaches the desired temperature.

Yields 4 servings.

Paleo Stew

This stew is filling, nutritious, and portable. Make enough to bring along to work, or even freeze it in single-serving bowls that you can carry with you. The vegetables used here are just a guideline—feel free to include whichever you like best.

- 1 pound beef, venison, or bison tips
- 2 cups organic tomato juice
- 2 cups water
- 1 yam, cubed into 1-inch pieces
- 1 cup carrots, sliced
- 1 cup kale, chopped
- 1 cup yellow onions, chunked
- 1 cup tomatoes, cubed
- 1 bay leaf
- 2 teaspoons unprocessed sea salt
- 1 sprig rosemary
- 1 teaspoon thyme

Sear your meat just to brown it a bit, and then toss all of your ingredients into a slow cooker.

Cook on low for 7–9 hours, or on high 3–5 hours.

Yields about 6 servings.

Garlic Broccoli

A great side dish or even a stand-alone snack, this recipe delivers good carbs, phytonutrients, and micronutrients galore. You can't go wrong!

- 2 cups broccoli florets
- 1 teaspoon extra-virgin olive oil
- 1 teaspoon garlic
- ⅛ teaspoon dried or fresh basil, chopped
- 1 pinch unprocessed sea salt
- 1 pinch cracked black pepper

Steam the broccoli as usual.

In a small skillet, heat the olive oil on medium, and sauté the garlic just until it starts to turn brown. Add the basil, salt, and pepper, and remove from heat.

Toss broccoli in the garlic oil and serve.

Yields 1 serving.

(12)

MEAL PLANS FOR SPECIFIC STRENGTH SPORTS

The primary variation in eating plans for endurance athletes competing in different sports is quantity of food. More than how often you eat, or what you eat, the amount that you eat is going to be determined by exactly how much stress you're putting on your body and how often you're doing it. As already discussed, the Paleo diet isn't about counting calories, it's about listening to your body and eating when you're hungry. That being said, strength training isn't exactly a typical activity in which our caveman ancestors would have participated.

Since your goal more often than not is to build lean muscle, you have to anticipate what your body will need before your belly starts to growl. That's okay, too—it just requires a different approach than typically followed. The following pages offer sample meal plans for various strength-training events.

Strength-Training Plan

This is probably the purest form of training because, though people who strength train certainly want to look good, their primary goal is to get stronger. The best way to do that is to work your muscles according to your approved training regimen and follow a clean diet providing plenty of protein and carbs so that your muscles can repair and get strong. Since you're not focusing on gaining mass, you can truly go with the Paleo theory of eating when you're hungry, as long as you eat well before and after you work out. Here is a good sample plan to get you started:

Breakfast 1–2 Hours Pre-Workout: Western Omelet Cup, 1 Banana Carrot Nut
Muffin, water

On the Go: Paleo Sports Drink (see Chapter 5), water

Immediate Post-Workout Recovery: Berrylicious Post-Workout Paleo Potion, lots of water

Post-Recovery Meal: Paleo Stew, water

Meal 5: Best-Ever Beef Kabobs, water

Body Building Plan

If you're trying to bulk up, you're going to be eating at least every two hours, and you'll need to
eat a good combination of proteins, carbs, and healthful fats in order to build muscle without
getting fat. Use your calipers to keep track of body fat as you gain, so this doesn't become an
issue. Here's a good sample of a day's worth of food for you:

Breakfast 1–2 Hours Pre-Workout: Egg-White Hash, 1 cup cantaloupe, Savory Sweet
Potato Hash Browns, 1 cup grapes, water

On the Go: Paleo Sports Drink, water

Immediate Post-Workout Recovery: Berrylicious Post-Workout Paleo Potion, lots of water

Post-Recovery Meal: Paleo Pesto Chicken (one piece), Garlic Broccoli, 1 cup
strawberries, water

Meal 5: Nutty Chopped Salad, water

Meal 6: Cajun Tilapia, Mashed Cauliflower, water

Meal 7: The second piece of Paleo Pesto Chicken, banana, Kale Succotash, water

CrossFit Workout Meal Plan

Much like strength training, CrossFit training doesn't require a specific diet other than that you make it healthful. You need to incorporate a wide range of foods and the correct ratio of proteins, complex carbohydrates, and healthful fats. Because it's a training program designed to meet a wide range of needs, from those of top military personnel to the elderly, dietary needs are going to vary widely. This is just a sample meal plan, so take it and adjust as you see fit.

Breakfast 1–2 Hours Pre-Workout: Paleo Waffles with Maple Syrup, 1/2 cup strawberries, water

On the Go: Paleo Sports Drink, water

Immediate Post-Workout Recovery: Berrylicious Post-Workout Paleo Potion, lots of water

Post-Recovery Meal: Mediterranean Salmon, Savory Sweet Potato Hash Browns, water

Meal 5: Nutty Chopped Salad, water

Meal 6: Cajun Tilapia, Mashed Cauliflower, water

Leaning-Out Meal Plan

If you're trying to get into competition shape, you want to lose as much fat as possible without compromising all of that muscle you've worked so hard to gain. You're going to be eating less, but do it right and start far enough in advance so that you can lose one and a half to two pounds per week and still meet your goal. Use your calipers as well as the scale to keep track of your loss: If you're losing muscle, it's a good sign that you're not eating enough, so adjust accordingly. Shoot for a calorie deficit but not a huge one.

Breakfast 1–2 Hours Pre-Workout: 2 Western Omelet Cups, 1 cup cantaloupe, water

On the Go: Paleo Sports Drink, water

Immediate Post-Workout Recovery: Berrylicious Post-Workout Paleo Potion, lots of water

Post-Recovery Meal: Best-Ever Beef Kabobs, Mashed Cauliflower, 1 cup strawberries, water

Meal 5: Egg-White Hash

Meal 6: Cajun Tilapia

Meal 7: Paleo Pesto Chicken, Garlic Broccoli

Meal 8: Leftover Beef Kabobs

Regardless of what your strength-training goals are, you need to feed your body sufficiently to recover. Lifting, especially heavy lifting, can seriously damage your muscles and cause permanent damage if you don't eat properly and train under the tutelage of a professional—at least until you get a good handle on how to train correctly. Building muscle and losing fat aren't quick; both goals take time and hard work to achieve. So set your goals, determine your priorities, and prepare to get in the best shape of your life!

Before closing things out, it seemed only fair to let you know that following a Paleo diet to meet your fitness goals doesn't mean you have to sacrifice the sweet stuff. In the next chapter, you'll learn how to whip up some decadent desserts, caveman-style!

(13)

ATHLETE-FRIENDLY DESSERTS

Two of the goals of the Paleo diet are to stop eating nutrient-poor processed foods and to break the sugar addiction that afflicts so many Western eaters. That doesn't mean you have to live the rest of your life without eating dessert. In fact, there are many decadent choices you can use to cure your sweet tooth and meet your carbohydrate needs, especially for pre-performance or night-before carb-loading. Remember, however, that dessert is meant to be a treat in an otherwise healthful-eating lifestyle.

You still can't eat sugar, flour, or any of the other harmful ingredients used in typical desserts, but trust us when we say you won't miss them! Before we move on to the recipes, let's talk about some ingredients you can use to make delicious treats packed with mostly healthful carbs, fats, and protein. Get ready for dessert, Paleo Athlete–style!

Honey

It's sweet, it's healthful, and it comes in a variety of flavors, depending upon what local ingredients are used. You always want to go with local honey because there's evidence to suggest that honey made from local plants can actually help you avoid allergies related to airborne pollens. It also has antimicrobial, antibacterial, and antifungal properties, which is why it was often used in poultices throughout history.

From a nutritive perspective, the glycemic index of one tablespoon of honey, particularly floral honey, is fairly low, and it has several different trace minerals as well as a small amount of protein. It's also a natural substance made by bees—rather than machines—so it falls squarely into the Paleo basket.

Maple Syrup

Pure maple syrup is one of the most overlooked, naturally delicious and nutritious foods ever. It has an extremely low-glycemic load and boasts several different minerals. As a matter of fact, one tablespoon of maple syrup contains about one-third of your daily requirement of manganese. It also has a good amount of omega-6 fatty acids.

Sweeteners to Avoid and Why

It may seem redundant to list sweeteners that you can't use, but sometimes it's helpful to know the reason instead of just being told, "Because it's not Paleo." That's no answer, so let's examine a couple of sweeteners that seem acceptable on the surface but really aren't:

- **Stevia:** Though it comes from a plant, the vast majority of stevia powders have chemical additives, and the syrups, unless marked organic, may contain pesticides. Also, this is a new product, and there aren't any long-term studies available to observe its effects.

- **Agave Syrup:** As with stevia, it's a natural plant, but that doesn't mean it doesn't contain pesticides. The main issue most Paleo eaters have with agave syrup, however, is that it's highly processed, sometimes using an enzymatic process, and that it contains concentrated fructose and the immune-stimulating toxin saponin, though probably in such small amounts in a teaspoon as to be negligible.

The key is to be sensible. If you believe that stevia or agave syrup is okay, then use it. For the sake of sticking as close to natural foods that Paleolithic man could have hunted, gathered, and immediately eaten (or cooked, then eaten), we're going to stick to honey and maple syrup.

Almond Flour vs. Almond Meal

The difference between almond flour and meal is that flour is finely ground, whereas meal is coarsely ground. This makes an enormous difference when baking, so be sure to use the product the recipe calls for. Since they're both made simply from ground almonds, they contain all of the same nutrients as the nut.

Finely ground (blanched) almond flour is fairly light compared to other nut flours and is substituted at a 1:1 ratio for wheat flours. It's great for crumbly or chewy baked goods like muffins, cookies, or crumb cakes. If you're using more wet ingredients, you may want to add in some coconut flour.

Coconut Flour

Coconut flour is extremely dense and full of fiber, so it absorbs liquids well. You need to use only a small amount, at least in comparison to what you're used to using in traditional baking. It's made by drying coconut pulp and grinding it up, so it will lend your dessert a slight coconut flavor and works especially nicely in recipes such as cakes and shortbread cookies that call for more wet ingredients. A rule of thumb is to substitute one-quarter the amount of coconut flour to wheat flour, but you may have to play with your particular brand a bit to get the right ratio.

Arrowroot Powder

Made from dried arrowroot, this is used to beef up your coconut flour recipes or to act as a thickening agent. It adds a nice lightness to your recipes and can be substituted 1:1 for cornstarch. Keep in mind, though, it's not effective as a binding agent.

Tapioca Starch/Flour

This isn't the same thing as arrowroot, though many people make that mistake. Tapioca is made from ground yucca root and is excellent as a thickener and to add elasticity to your recipes. It also gives a bit more spring to your cakes and acts as a binding agent. You can substitute it for wheat flour at a 1:1 ratio, but it's better for health and textural reasons to use in conjunction with other Paleo flours.

Though there are other nut, fruit, and vegetable flours available, these are the most commonly used flours, thickeners, and sweeteners in Paleo recipes. Now that you have a general idea of some basic ingredients, let's make something sweet!

Single Caveman Microwave Brownie

This is a great single-serving brownie recipe that's perfect to make on the fly, or if you're just craving something sweet right now. It takes only about four minutes to prepare, start to finish, and is made in a coffee mug in the microwave.

- 2 tablespoons pure cocoa powder
- 3 tablespoons almond flour
- 1 tablespoon almond butter
- 1 tablespoon light maple syrup
- 1 egg
- 1 pinch unprocessed sea salt

Add all ingredients to a microwave mug and stir well.

Microwave for 2 minutes and enjoy!

Yields 1 serving.

Coconut Crumb Cake

This cake is sure to hit the spot if you're looking for that after-dinner bite to cure your sweet tooth. It's perfect for that night-before meal to add some carbs to your store before the big event.

- ½ cup almond flour
- ⅓ cup coconut flour
- ¼ teaspoon unprocessed sea salt
- 1½ teaspoons baking powder
- 1 teaspoon baking soda
- 1 teaspoon cinnamon

- 4 whole eggs
- 1 cup full-fat coconut milk
- ¼ cup honey + 2 tablespoons
- ¼ cup toasted almonds, slivered
- ¼ cup coconut, shredded

Preheat oven to 350 degrees F.

In a large mixing bowl, combine all of your dry ingredients except for the slivered almonds and shredded coconut, and then add your wet ingredients except for the extra 2 tablespoons of honey. Mix for 1 minute or until thoroughly combined.

Pour into a greased 8 x 8 inch cake pan, and bake 25 minutes or until the edges brown.

Remove from oven and sprinkle the almonds and coconut over top, then drizzle over them the last 2 tablespoons of honey.

Allow to cool and serve.

Yields 8 servings.

Paleo Apple Crisp

This stuff is so good you'll be transported back to grandma's kitchen. It's high carb but doesn't have any of that bad-for-you, refined white stuff that leaves you feeling too bloated to compete.

- 2 Granny Smith apples, peeled and cored
- 1 tablespoon raisins
- 2 tablespoons maple syrup (light is nice but any will do)
- 2 teaspoons cinnamon
- ¼ teaspoon ground cloves
- 2 tablespoons course almond meal
- 1 tablespoon honey
- 1 tablespoon butter or coconut oil, melted
- ¼ cup water

Preheat oven to 350 degrees F.

Place apples, raisins, maple syrup, cinnamon, and cloves in a small bowl, and toss to coat.

In a separate small dish, combine almond meal, honey, and butter or oil, and mix together to make a crumble.

Put apple mixture in a small soufflé dish, and add water. Then top with the crumble.

Bake for 25 minutes or until apples are tender, water is evaporated, and crumble is brown.

Yields 1 serving.

Maple Cream Fudge

This old-fashioned dessert is definitely high-carb and pairs especially well with a cup of after-dinner coffee. Rich, creamy, and decadent, this treat is also great for a quick burst of energy.

- 2 cups maple syrup
- 1 tablespoon honey
- ¾ cup almond milk or heavy cream
- 1 teaspoon unprocessed sea salt

If you're not an old hand at candy making, you'll need a candy thermometer here in order to produce exactly the proper consistency.

In a medium, heavy-bottomed pan, combine the syrup, honey, and milk/cream.

Stir well and attach the candy thermometer to the side of the pan, making sure that it isn't touching the bottom. Cook over medium heat, stirring frequently until a small ball of the mixture placed in cold water is soft and pliable. Don't scrape the sides of the pan.

Allow to cool for about 3 minutes, and then pour into your stand mixer and beat for 7 minutes or until the candy loses its glass and is opaque.

Spread into a greased loaf pan, and sprinkle sea salt on top.

Allow to set, cut into 2-inch squares, and enjoy.

Yields about 10 pieces.

Sweet Potato Gingerbread Cupcakes with Maple Frosting

This sumptuous treat is great for when you're on the go or if you want to celebrate a particularly awesome workout. Don't let the large number of ingredients turn you off to making these—they're definitely worth the effort.

- 1 cup sweet potato, pureed
- 2 whole eggs
- 1 teaspoon vanilla
- ½ cup almond butter
- 1 cup almond flour
- 1 teaspoon baking soda
- 2 teaspoons baking powder
- 1 tablespoon pumpkin pie spice
- ½ cup coconut butter (for frosting)
- ½ cup organic coconut oil (for frosting)
- 3 tablespoons medium to dark maple syrup (for frosting)
- ½ teaspoon vanilla extract (for frosting)

Preheat oven to 350 degrees F, and line your muffin pan with cupcake papers.

Mix sweet potato puree, eggs, vanilla, and almond butter in a medium bowl.

In a separate bowl, combine dry ingredients and add to sweet potato mixture. Blend well for about 2 minutes, then fill cupcake papers two-thirds full.

Bake 25–30 minutes or until toothpick comes out clean.

Place on cooling rack and make your icing. Simply mix together the coconut butter, coconut oil, maple syrup, and vanilla. When cupcakes are cool, ice them and enjoy.

Yields 12 cupcakes.

(14)

ANYTIME SNACKS FOR ATHLETES

One of the most important parts of maintaining a healthy body is fueling it properly, but sometimes that's hard to do. Especially when you're training, you need to eat at least every couple of hours, but when you're going to school or working, making that happen can be difficult.

Even if you're a stay-at-home parent or you work from home, it can be tough to cook a meal that often, so the following healthful snacks are a great option for those hectic times and will keep you going. Then there are those moments you're just looking for something to munch on but want to avoid potato chips with ranch dip. These tasty recipes have got you covered there, too!

Super Simple Trail Mix

Packed with a combination of good carbs and protein, this blend will keep you moving until you can get in a real meal. The crunchy saltiness will ease your craving as well as help your body restore lost electrolytes.

- ¼ cup almonds
- ¼ cup cashews
- ¼ cup pecans, quartered
- ¼ cup coconut flakes
- ¼ cup dried pineapple
- ¼ cup dates, chopped
- ¼ cup dried bananas
- 1 pinch unprocessed sea salt

Mix all ingredients in a small bowl, and toss well to combine.

Store in an airtight container—if it lasts that long!

Yields 1¾ cups.

Cajun Sweet Potato Chips

If you're looking for crispy, salty, and satisfying, then these chips are for you. We'll even go so far as to say that they taste way better than the saturated, fat-laden, plain old potato chips. Try them and see!

- 2 sweet potatoes, sliced extra thin
- 2 tablespoons coconut oil, melted
- ¼ teaspoon Cajun seasoning (see Cajun Tilapia in Chapter 10)

Preheat oven to 400 degrees F.

Place sweet potatoes in a medium bowl, and drizzle coconut oil over them. Sprinkle with Cajun seasoning and toss to coat.

Layer on a parchment paper–lined cookie sheet, and bake 10 minutes or until chips are crisp.

Yields 4 servings.

Spinach Artichoke Dip

Creamy and flavorful, this nutritious dip is terrific with Cajun Sweet Potato Chips or your favorite veggies—it makes you feel good about eating right.

- 1 box frozen organic spinach
- 1 (14-ounce) jar of artichoke hearts
- 2 teaspoons extra-virgin olive oil
- 2 garlic cloves, minced
- 2 scallions, chopped
- 2 teaspoons lemon juice
- ½ teaspoon onion powder
- ½ teaspoon garlic powder
- ½ teaspoon unprocessed sea salt
- ¼ teaspoon cracked black pepper
- 1 cup cream cheese or cashew cream

Drain and chop the spinach and artichokes.

Warm the olive oil in a medium skillet on low heat, and sauté the garlic and scallions for about 1 minute.

Add in the spinach, artichoke, lemon juice, and spices, and heat until hot.

Add the cream cheese or cashew cream, and stir till combined.

Yields about 2 cups.

Cucumber Turkey Sammies

These crunchy little crowd pleasers will be a hit with all of your friends and family, regardless of whether they're eating healthfully or not. Packed with antioxidants and protein, they're sure to be a staple snack.

- 5 slices of turkey breast cut in half
- 5 cherry tomatoes, halved
- ½ avocado, peeled, cored, and sliced
- 10 cucumber slices, ½-inch thick and cut lengthwise
- 3 red onion rings, chopped

This one's really simple. Just place 1 slice of turkey breast, tomato, and avocado on each of 5 slices of cucumber.

Sprinkle onions over them, and top with another slice of cucumber.

Yields 5 sammies.

Paleo Ice Treats

Though these popsicles taste sugary and fruity, they actually pack quite a nutritious punch. They make an excellent post-workout treat, helping you to replace lost electrolytes and get rehydrated.

- 2 cups strawberries
- 1 cup sour cherries, pitted
- 2 bananas
- ½ cup frozen spinach
- 1 cup apple juice

Six-ounce yogurt cups are the perfect tool for this job, and you can buy ice treat sticks at your local craft store or department store. If you can't find them, just freeze your puree in the yogurt cups, and eat them with a spoon.

Put all ingredients in the blender, and mix until smooth.

Pour into molds or yogurt cups and freeze.

Yields about 6 treats.

CONCLUSION

Hopefully you've found everything you need here to get you started on your path to Paleo eating. Choosing the right diet with a balanced blend of macronutrients can be tough, especially for athletes who like to take fitness to the next level. Your body has vastly different nutritional needs to repair your tissues, build new muscle, and keep you going throughout your workout, but the Paleo diet meets those needs in all respects.

As you've learned, the Paleo diet isn't actually a "diet": it's a way of life that focuses on eating healthful meals and staying active while avoiding foods that contain toxins that slowly poison us one way or another. Certainly, that's just a smart way to live regardless of your physical fitness goals. Lean proteins, quality carbs, and healthful fats are simply a recipe for good, disease-free living, and that's exactly what the Paleo diet prescribes.

Athletes know better than anyone that there is no such thing as a shortcut, magic pill, or surgical procedure that can instantly make you stacked and healthy—that requires months or even years of work, both at the gym and at the dinner table. The old saying, "You are what you eat," still applies today, so for those moments when you lose focus and are tempted by that huge slice of pizza, just keep that in mind. In short, your body is quite literally built one bite at a time.

So now you have the tools in hand; good luck on your Paleo-eating journey to health and fitness!

GLOSSARY

Aerobic exercise—Exercise such as walking, running, swimming, and cycling that elevates your heart rate and uses large muscles, while depending upon oxygen-generated energy from carbohydrates and fats to meet your exercise needs and keep your muscles energized. Aerobic exercise can be maintained for long periods of time, depending upon fitness level and cardiovascular health.

Almond flour—Gluten-free flour used in place of wheat flour in baking and cooking. It's made simply by grinding almonds into a fine flour.

Anaerobic exercise—High-intensity exercise such as lifting weights that burns through oxygen-generated energy from carbohydrate supplies faster than your body can replace it. This leads to muscle fatigue and promotes the destruction of old tissue so that new muscle can be built. The primary fuel source during anaerobic exercise is glucose.

Anabolic state—When your body uses food sources for energy instead of stores found in your tissues. Constantly fueling your body allows it to build muscle and repair tissue damaged during exercise.

Antinutrients—Compounds that inhibit the absorption of nutrients in your body. These include lipase, amylase, phytic acid, oxalic acid (oxylates), glucosinolates, and even some proteins such as gluten found in grains, trypsin inhibitors, and lectins found in legumes. Flavonoids are also antinutrients. Some of these, such as flavonoids, have positive functions as well, while others simply block absorption and even stimulate an inflammatory immune response.

BCAAs—Short for "branch chain amino acids," these are the protein building blocks that your body uses to build lean muscle.

Catabolic state—When your body runs out of food sources to use as fuel, and it begins to break down essential fat stores and muscle tissue for energy.

Coconut aminos—Derived from the coconut tree, this dark, tasty liquid is often used to replace soy sauce in recipes. It contains seventeen amino acids and has less than half the sodium of soy sauce.

Dilutional hyponatremia—Also known as water intoxication, this happens when you drink too much water without having balanced electrolytes. This is why it's so important to drink or eat foods that contain sodium, potassium, and magnesium if you're participating in exercise that causes salt and fluid loss.

Glycemic index—A number that determines how quickly a particular food raises blood glucose levels after you eat it. Specifically, the GI estimates how much one gram of available carbohydrate raises blood glucose level. As a comparison, straight glucose is 100. The bad thing about using the GI is that it doesn't factor in how much of the food you eat. It tells you only how much one gram affects you.

Glycemic load—A number that determines how much a food will raise blood glucose levels after eating it. One unit of glycemic load is equal to the effects of one gram of pure glucose. This measurement is easier to use than the glycemic index because it multiplies the GI by the carb content of the serving size that you're eating.

Hardgainer—A person who has difficulty putting on weight and muscle due to an extremely fast, efficient metabolism.

Homeostasis—Your body's tendency to maintain a balanced state. This includes pH, electrolytes, and any other function crucial to survival. Your body will pull from one area, such as muscles and tissue, in order to maintain a homeostatic state.

Macronutrients—Major nutrients your body needs in order to function properly and create energy. The three major macronutrients for the human body are fat, protein, and carbohydrates.

Micronutrients—Nutrients your body needs in small quantities to facilitate critical functions and physiological responses.

Muscle hypertrophy—An increase in the size of the cells that make up your muscles. Sarcoplasmic hypertrophy involves increasing the size of the muscle without focusing on strength.

Ursolic acid—A chemical found in apple peels, and in lesser quantities in cranberries, basil, bilberries, peppermint, rosemary, lavender, oregano, thyme, and prunes, which not only prevents muscle waste, but actually helps muscles grow. It's also rumored to be helpful with some types of cancer, but the research is still preliminary.

Made in the USA
San Bernardino, CA
12 May 2018